Endovascular Treatment of Aortic Aneurysms

Standard and Advanced Techniques

Endovascular Treatment of Aortic Aneurysms

Standard and Advanced Techniques

KONSTANTINOS P. DONAS, MD
Professor of Vascular Surgery
Consultant Vascular Surgeon
Department of Vascular Surgery
St. Franziskus Hospital Münster
Münster, Germany

GIOVANNI TORSELLO, MD
Professor of Vascular Surgery
Director of Clinic of Vascular and Endovascular Surgery, University of Münster
Chief of Department of Vascular Surgery, St. Franziskus Hospital Münster, Münster, Germany
Universitätsklinikum Münster
Waldeyerstraße, Münster, Germany

KENNETH OURIEL, MD
Professor of Vascular Surgery
CEO Syntactx
New York, NY, United States

ELSEVIER

ELSEVIER

3251 Riverport Lane
St. Louis, Missouri 63043

ENDOVASCULAR TREATMENT OF AORTIC ANEURYSMS:
STANDARD AND ADVANCED TECHNIQUES

ISBN: 978-0-323-51148-3

Content Strategist: Kayla Wolfe
Content Development Manager: Lucia Gunzel
Content Development Specialist: Kristen Helm
Publishing Services Manager: Deepthi Unni
Project Manager: Janish Ashwin Paul
Designer: Gopalakrishnan Venkatraman

Last digit is the print number: 9 8 7 6 5 4 3 2 1

To my beautiful young children, Pericles and Amalia, who spent a few hours less with me each day as I prepared and edited this book with the distinguish co-Editors and authors.

Konstantinos P. Donas

List of Contributors

Editors

Konstantinos P. Donas, MD
Professor of Vascular Surgery
Consultant Vascular Surgeon
Department of Vascular Surgery
St. Franziskus Hospital Münster
Hohenzollernring, Münster, Germany

Giovanni Torsello, MD
Professor of Vascular Surgery
Director of Clinic of Vascular and Endovascular Surgery, University of Münster
Chief of Department of Vascular Surgery, St. Franziskus Hospital Münster, Münster, Germany
Universitätsklinikum Münster
Waldeyerstraße, Münster, Germany

Kenneth Ouriel, MD
Professor of Vascular Surgery
CEO Syntactx
New York, NY, United States

Authors

Martin Austermann, MD
Assistant Professor of Vascular Surgery
Senior Consultant Vascular Surgeon
Department of Vascular Surgery
St. Franziskus Hospital Münster
Münster, Germany

Efthymios Beropoulis, MD
Fellow
Department of Vascular Surgery
St. Franziskus Hospital Münster
Münster, Germany

Theodosios Bisdas, MD
Assistant Professor of Vascular Surgery
Consultant Vascular Surgeon
Department of Vascular Surgery
St. Franziskus Hospital Münster
Münster, Germany

Michel Bosiers, MD
Vascular Surgeon
Department of Vascular Surgery
St. Franziskus Hospital Münster
Münster, Germany

Emiliano Chisci, MD
Consultant Vascular Surgeon
Clinic of Vascular Surgery
University of Florence
Florence, Italy
Department of Surgery
Vascular and Endovascular Surgery Unit
"San Giovanni di Dio" Hospital
Florence, Italy

Frank J. Criado, MD
Vascular Surgeon and Endovascular Specialist
MedStar Union Memorial Hospital
Baltimore, MD
Professor of Vascular Surgery
Baltimore University Hospital
Baltimore, MD

Konstantinos P. Donas, MD
Professor of Vascular Surgery
Consultant Vascular Surgeon
Department of Vascular Surgery
St. Franziskus Hospital Münster
Münster, Germany

Markus Eisenack, MD
Fellow
Clinic of Vascular and Endovascular Surgery
University of Münster
Münster, Germany

Stefano Fazzini, MD, PhD
Department of Vascular Surgery
San Filippo Neri Hospital
Rome, Italy

Mario Lachat, MD
Professor of Vascular Surgery
Clinic of Cardiovascular Surgery
University Hospital Zurich
Zurich, Switzerland

Francisco Marques de Azevedo
Head of Vascular and Endovascular Nurse Team in the OR
St. Franziskus Hospital
Münster, Germany

Stefano Michelagnoli, MD
Professor Vascular Surgeon
Clinic of Vascular Surgery
University of Florence
Florence, Italy

Kenneth Ouriel, MD
Professor of Vascular Surgery
CEO Syntactx
New York, NY, United States

Giuseppe Panuccio, MD
Consultant Vascular Surgeon
Clinic of Vascular and Endovascular Surgery
University of Münster
Münster, Germany

Johannes Schäfers, MD
Fellow
Clinic of Vascular and Endovascular Surgery
University of Münster
Münster, Germany

Arne Schwindt, MD
Consultant Vascular Surgeon
Department of Vascular Surgery
St. Franziskus Hospital Münster
Münster, Germany

Giovanni Federico Torsello, MD, BA
Fellow in Radiology
Institute of Diagnostic and Interventional Radiology and Nuclear Medicine
Charité–University Medicine Berlin
Berlin, Germany

Giovanni Torsello, MD
Professor of Vascular Surgery
Director of Clinic of Vascular and Endovascular Surgery, University of Münster
Chief of Department of Vascular Surgery, St. Franziskus Hospital Münster, Münster, Germany
Universitätsklinikum Münster
Waldeyerstraße, Münster, Germany

Nicola Troisi, MD
Consultant Vascular Surgeon
Clinic of Vascular Surgery
University of Florence
Florence, Italy
Department of Surgery
Vascular and Endovascular Surgery Unit
San Giovanni di Dio Hospital
Florence, Italy

Foreword

We think of abdominal aortic aneurysm repair as an "old technique." However, even endovascular aneurysm repair (EVAR) has been in existence for more than 25 years. In fact, we have merely scratched the surface of possibilities for the efficient treatment of the broad spectrum of aortic aneurysmal disease. Open surgical modalities have been relegated to those patients in whom current endovascular technology is inadequate to achieve a safe and effective aortic repair. At present, open surgery is limited to patients with proximal neck characteristics incompatible with long-term, durable fixation and seal, while maintaining perfusion to the renal and visceral vessels. To a lesser extent, atherosclerotic and aneurysmal iliac artery disease also limits the use of endovascular modalities. Occasionally, iliac anatomic issues impede safe EVAR.

Advanced endovascular techniques for aortic aneurysm repair developed in this clinical landscape, where the universe of aneurysms suitable for endovascular repair remains short of uniform. Advanced techniques evolved to expand the range of aortic aneurysm disease treatable without open surgery. Proximal neck issues were addressed in a manner following the lead of open surgery, reaching to higher, more proximal levels in the aorta and relying on aortic segments free from aneurysmal degeneration. The parallels to open surgical treatment of proximal aortic aneurysms are unmistakable. Just as traditional open surgical procedures adopted the use of the retroperitoneal approach, supravisceral aortic clamping, and renal-visceral-intercostal artery reimplantation for such aneurysms, so too has endovascular therapy progressed.

Adjunctive parallel grafts, stents, fenestrations, and branch grafts have become important endovascular adjuncts, each designed so that more proximal aspects of the repair might be based on normal aorta. As with complex open surgical repair of proximal aortic aneurysms, the technical aspects of advanced EVAR can be elusive to practitioners. The advanced skills necessary to repair juxtarenal, suprarenal, and thoracoabdominal aortic aneurysms may be unfamiliar to the occasional interventionist, just as the open surgical techniques for such aneurysms are far from common. Similarly, management of the tight aortic bifurcation, iliac artery atherosclerotic disease, and common iliac aneurysms each represents challenges to the endovascular practitioner. Failure to adequately identify, plan for, and address such anatomic issues can result in immediate occlusive and hemorrhagic complications and long-term patency issues.

The genesis of this book was to provide the practicing endovascular clinician with a state-of-the-art reference for the current thought process in the endovascular treatment of *complex aortic aneurysms*, briefly defined as those aneurysms that defy treatment with standard, off-the-shelf endograft technology. Prior to embarking on novel techniques to address unusual anatomy, however, the clinician must be well grounded in the endovascular treatment of standard abdominal aortic aneurysms. For this reason, the text begins with an introduction to infrarenal endovascular repair, including pre- and postoperative patient management. The chapters then describe modifications of standard techniques so that challenging iliac access can be safely addressed and hostile proximal neck characteristics can be recognized and treated. Of necessity, the text flows into the use of advanced techniques to preserve renal and visceral artery perfusion for more proximally oriented aneurysms, with chapters covering a broad range of techniques, including chimneys, fenestrations, and for thoracoabdominal and arch aneurysms, branch grafts and hybrid endovascular-open surgical approaches. The management of endoleaks is discussed as the most frequent early and late complication of any endovascular repair. Advanced intraprocedural imaging techniques, specifically fusion imaging, is addressed, recognizing the interdependence of radiologic visualization and endovascular outcome, as well as the increasing importance of minimizing radiation exposure to the patient, surgeon, and procedural staff.

No book can replace the tried-and-true, time-honored method of hands-on surgical training. No words in a paragraph, no images on a page, and no emeritus surgeon cobbling together a foreword can substitute for the intensive, second-to-second, tactile and visual experiences of live surgical training. This volume is not designed to replace the traditional teaching paradigm, and the reader should be cautioned that this text cannot substitute for the apprenticeship model so essential to the acquisition of endovascular skills. Still, this book provides the endovascular neophyte with a foundation for the clinical study of endovascular aortic technology. For the master endovascular technician, this textbook will at least remind the practitioner of novel techniques that might be employed in the "next case." Also, the chapters may stimulate the development of even more innovative, yet undiscovered procedures—procedures that will enhance patient care to maximize safety and more effectively treat the multifaceted continuum of aortic aneurysmal disease.

Kenneth Ouriel, MD
Professor of Vascular Surgery
CEO syntactx
New York, NY

Preface

Until a few years ago, open surgery was the only form of treatment for patients with aortic pathologies. However, less invasive methods, such as endografting with standard, chimney, branched, and fenestrated stent-grafts, have been increasing in importance. Additionally, the sustained number of high-risk patients has led to a shift toward endovascular techniques.

This book focuses on illustrating standard and advanced alternative techniques to open surgery for the treatment of aortic aneurysms. The reported cases have been treated in the Department of Vascular Surgery at St. Franziskus Hospital Münster, Germany. All possible approaches are described in a step-by-step manner, including limitations of the presented techniques and a review of the most relevant literature.

The information in this text is based on our clinical experience of many years and may not always align with recommendations of the device manufacturers. In this context, alternative approaches to the presented techniques may be feasible and successful, especially because some techniques (e.g., use of fenestrated grafts) were introduced more than 15 years ago, and others (e.g., chimney technique) can be performed with several abdominal and covered endovascular devices. Our main goal, however, is to present the techniques as performed at our institution in a standardized and uniform manner.

Since thoracoabdominal or arch aortic aneurysms still represent one of the most demanding pathologies, with high morbidity and mortality, even in specialized cardiovascular centers, the description of the complete endovascular approach with sandwich techniques or branched endografts has a central role in this volume.

We hope that this book will be helpful to your daily clinical practice in choosing successful, patient-oriented endovacular treatment of aortic aneurysms.

Giovanni Torsello, MD
Professor of Vascular Surgery
Director of Clinic of Vascular and Endovascular Surgery
University of Münster
Chief of Department of Vascular Surgery
St. Franziskus Hospital Münster
Münster, Germany

Contents

CHAPTER 1

The Percutaneous Approach of Endovascular Aortic Aneurysm Repair

MARKUS EISENACK • KONSTANTINOS P. DONAS

The endovascular treatment of aortic aneurysms is based on stent-graft delivery through the common femoral artery (CFA). The procedure has evolved over the years. Since the development of the percutaneous approach in the late 1990s, several surveys have been performed and have promoted the advantages of this technique.[1-4] The percutaneous approach was associated with a shorter time to ambulation and fewer complications compared with an open cutdown to the groin vessels, including a reduced risk of events such as wound infection, lymphocele, and hematomas.[5]

All currently available closure devices are approved for use only up to 10-French (10F) sheath sizes.[6] With the introduction of the "preclose" technique, however, it was possible to close access vessels after endovascular aneurysm repair (EVAR), which requires larger-bore sheaths.[7]

The Prostar XL 10F device (Abbott Laboratories. Abbott Park, Illinois, USA) consists of four components (Fig. 1.1). The first two components are a hydrophilic catheter for guiding the system into the aorta and a marker lumen for identification of correct device position in the vessel (Fig. 1.2). The third component is a sheath containing four lancelike nitinol needles, which are connected to two braided sutures (Fig. 1.3). The fourth component is a rotating barrel for dissection and needle capture. The device is advanced into the artery to guide the needle trajectory through the subcutaneous tissue, with the sutures being pulled out from the inside through the arterial wall (Figs. 1.4 and 1.5).

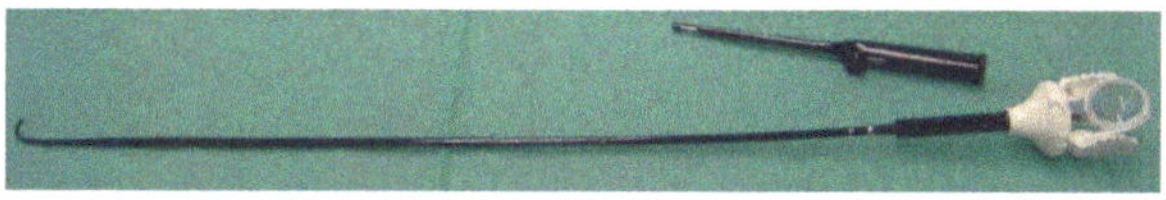

FIG. 1.1 The Prostar XL 10F device.

PRECLOSE TECHNIQUE

After puncture of the CFA and insertion of an 8F short sheath, and with careful blunt dissection of the subcutaneous tissue down to the vessel wall with a mosquito clamp, the Prostar XL 10F is advanced and deployed. The sutures are fixed loosely with a small clamp, and a 14F sheath replaces the closure system. After deployment of the stent-graft, the sutures are tied to the vessel with a fisherman's knot (Fig. 1.6).

To avoid major blood loss in case of a failed closure, a guidewire is left in place and maintains access to the vessel. Hemorrhage is controlled during dissection of the groin and exposure of the vessel. If oozing occurs after securing the knots, these should be held against the vessel wall with the knot pusher for several minutes, manually compressing the artery above the puncture site (Fig. 1.7).

If compression is not effective, a polytetrafluoroethylene (PTFE) felt pledget can be sewn with the four vascular sutures of the Prostar device to achieve hemostasis. The wound is closed using a topical liquid skin adhesive.

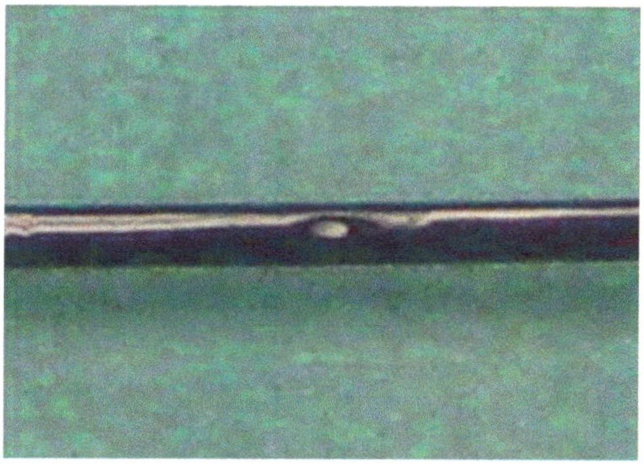

FIG. 1.2 The marker lumen of the Prostar device.

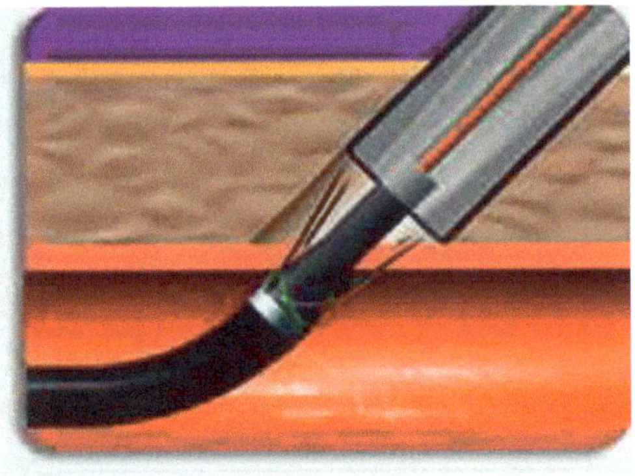

FIG. 1.3 The lancelike nitinol needles are crossed and connected to two braided sutures.

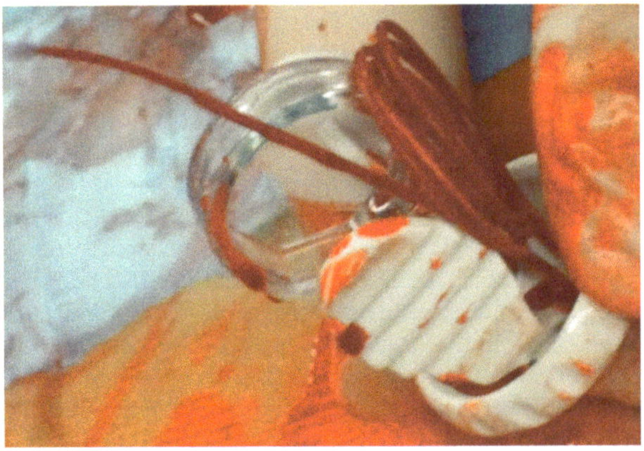

FIG. 1.4 Rotating barrel for insertion in the femoral artery. The correct position of the Prostar device in the femoral artery is confirmed by backbleeding.

LITERATURE REVIEW

The largest single-center series on the Prostar device was from Münster, Germany.[8] Between January 2004 and December 2005, 535 consecutive patients were treated for aneurysmal disease of the aorta by endovascular means and percutaneous approach. No patient was excluded because of obesity, severe calcification of the CFA, previous interventions, or operations in the groin. The failure rate was correlated with risk factors that included obesity (body mass index [BMI] >35), extensive calcification of the CFA, previous interventions or scars in the groin, and experience of the surgeon ("experienced" defined by more than 30 closures performed with Prostar XL). Primary success was achieved in 96.1% (n = 868 groins) of all percutaneous approaches. Secondary procedures were performed in 35 cases (3.9%) to treat insufficient bleeding control (28), false aneurysm (4), or arterial thrombosis (3). In 23 cases the complications were treated by open-vessel exposure and direct suture repair. In the remaining 12 patients the failure was corrected using a PTFE pledget sutured with the Prostar sutures. The access complications were detected and treated during the first week after EVAR in all cases; no patients presented with late complications. No wound complications were recorded during the early or late period.

An assessment of factors predictive of complications identified severe calcification of the CFA (37.8%), scar in the groin (23.8%), or EVAR by a surgeon with experience of less than 30 percutaneous cases (14%). The presence of a scar in the groin also correlated with the necessity of late conversion to open femoral artery repair (P <0.001). The development of false aneurysms occurred significantly more

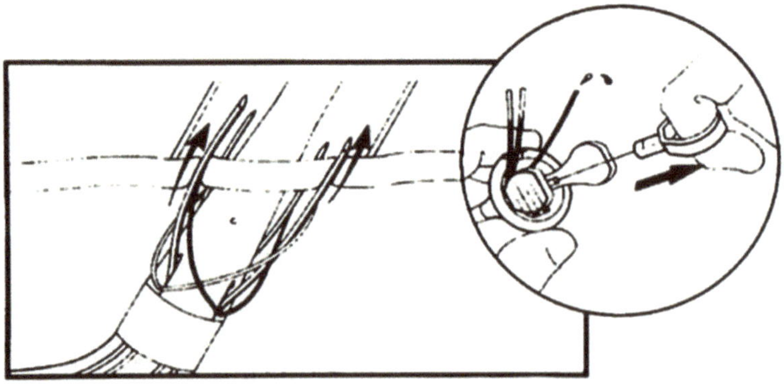

FIG. 1.5 The sutures are pulled through the arterial wall.

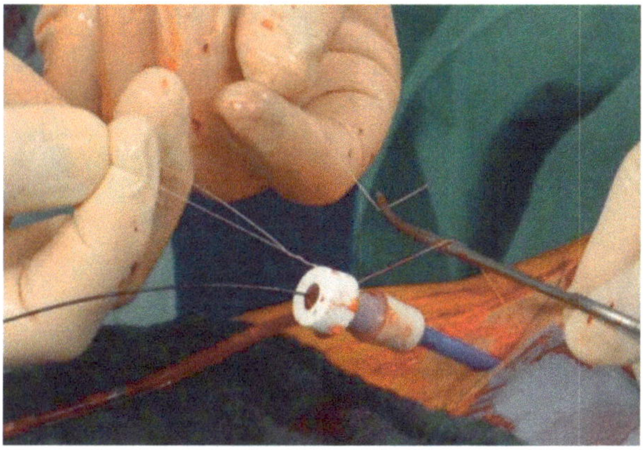

FIG. 1.6 The fisherman's knot technique.

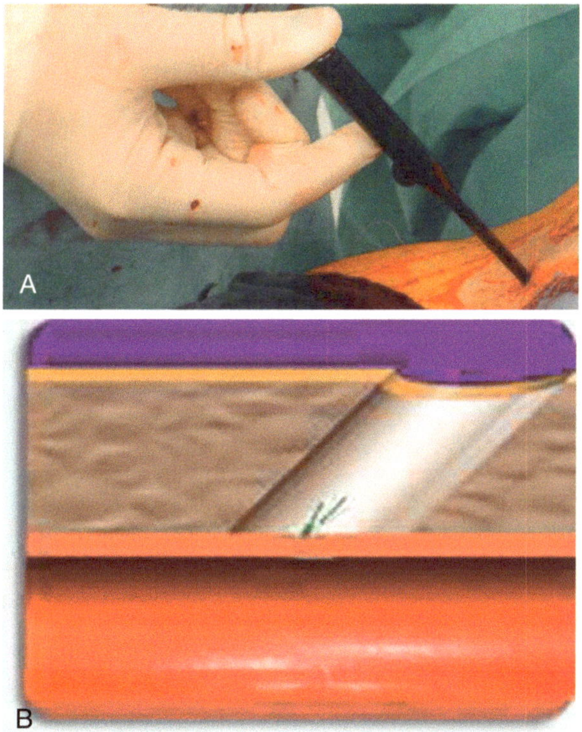

FIG. 1.7 **A, B,** Compression of the artery above the puncture site by the knot pusher.

often in scarred groins (P <0.05). Sheath size and scar in the groin also correlated with early conversion, but to a much lesser degree (respectively, P <0.05). Obesity was not a risk factor for any complication.

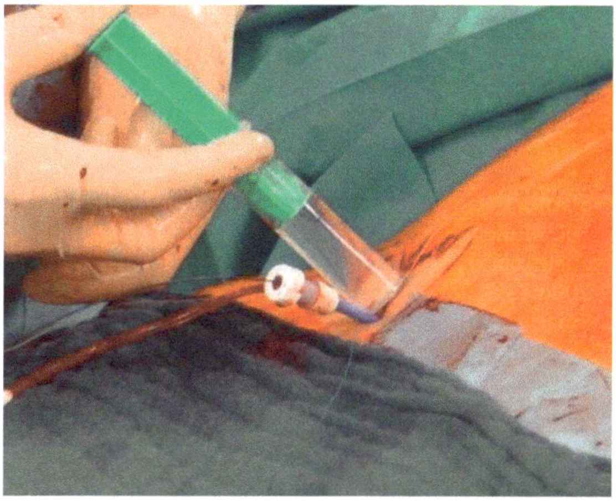

FIG. 1.8 In obese patients, systematic flushing of the groin and, after insertion of the Prostar device, flushing of the port exclude mechanical obstruction of the marker lumen.

Percutaneous treatment of obese patients has the advantage of reducing wound complications but requires precise dissection of the subcutaneous tissue to advance the device down to the vessel. Backbleeding through the marker lumen of the Prostar device must be observed to confirm sufficient penetration of the catheter into the lumen. We recommend flushing the groin (Fig. 1.8) and the port and slightly rotating the device to exclude mechanical obstruction of the marker lumen.

A prospective randomized study evaluating results of the surgical cutdown versus the percutaneous technique indicated a lower access site complication rate in the percutaneous group.[5] Avoiding an open surgical femoral artery exposure was preferable to the patient and decreased the rate of wound infection and lymph fistula.

SUMMARY

Use of the Prostar XL 10F system for vascular closure after EVAR is safe and effective. Surgeon experience is one of the most significant predictors of success. Anterior wall calcification of the CFA and scarring of the groin are predictors of primary failure, whereas obesity and sheath size do not appear to affect outcome. Repair of the artery when percutaneous access fails is usually not difficult. Proper training and handling of the device are key to treatment success.

REFERENCES

1. Howell M, Doughtery K, Strickman N, Krajcer Z. Percutanous repair of abdominal aortic aneurysms using the Aneurx stent graft and the percutaneous vascular surgery device. *Cathet Cardiovasc Intervent*. 2002;55:281–287.
2. Starnes BW, Anderson CA, Ronsivalle JA, Stockmaster NR, Mullenix PS, Statler JD. Totally percutaneous aortic aneurysm repair: Experience and prudence. *J Vasc Surg*. 2006;43:270–276.
3. Singh N, Adams E, Neville R, Deaton DH. Percutaneous endovascular AAA repair. *Endovasc Today*. 2005:39–44.
4. Can A, Torsello G, Umscheid T. The arterial approaches for endovascular aortic grafting. Endovascular aortic repair: The State of The Art. In: Branchereau A, Jacobs M, eds. Oxford: Blackwell Publishing; 2008:57–61.
5. Torsello GB, Kasprzak B, Klenk E, Tessarek J, Osada N, Torsello GF. Endovascular suture versus cutdown for endovascular aneurysm repair: A prospective randomized pilot study. *J Vasc Surg*. 2003;38:78–82.
6. Jean-Baptiste E, Hassen-Khodja R, Haudebourg P, Bouillanne PJ, Declemy S, Batt M. Percutaneous closure devices for endovascular repair of infrarenal aortic aneurysms: A prospective, non-randomized comparative study. *Eur J Vasc Endovasc Surg*. 2008;35:422–428.
7. Traul DK, Clair DG, Gray B, O'Hara PJ, Ouriel K. Percutaneous endovascular repair of infrarenal abdominal aortic aneurysms: A feasibility study. *J Vasc Surg*. 2000;32:770–776.
8. Eisenack M, Umscheid T, Tessarek J, Torsello GF, Torsello GB. Percutaneous endovascular aortic aneurysm repair: a prospective evaluation of safety, efficiency, and risk factors. *J Endovasc Ther*. 2009 Dec;16(6):708–713.

CHAPTER 2

The Standard Endovascular Aneurysm Repair Procedure

KONSTANTINOS P. DONAS

Since the first publication of endovascular aneurysm repair (EVAR) by Volodos et al.[1] and Parodi et al.,[2] a remarkable evolution in device design, components, and delivery systems has ushered in the applicability of EVAR to challenging anatomies. The main goals remain the optimization of the apposition of the proximal stent-graft to the aortic wall and the improvement of the system's ability to track through hostile iliac anatomies, as occurs in cases of severe calcification and angulation.

PROCEDURAL STEPS

The Endurant stent-graft system (Medtronic, Santa Rosa, California, USA) was designed to overcome anatomic limitations, expanding the EVAR population suitable for endovascular repair. The Endurant device is the primary abdominal endograft for infrarenal abdominal aortic aneurysms (AAAs) in Münster, Germany, centers. The short, proximal M-shaped stents, the absence of a longitudinal bar, and the hydrophilic coating of the delivery system represent notable features of this latest-generation endograft. The device received Conformité Européenne (CE) mark approval in July 2008.

The EVAR procedure consists of five steps:

1. After bilateral puncture of the common femoral artery, 8-French (8F) sheaths are inserted in each groin with the Seldinger technique; 5000 units of heparin is administered. In addition, bilateral femoral placement of the Prostar system allows percutaneous access and closure (see Chapter 1).
2. The Terumo wire is inserted in the descending aorta and a pigtail catheter advanced over the aortic arch and into the ascending aorta. This is followed by insertion of the Lunderquist double-curved stiff wire into the ascending aorta. The contralateral side will be used for angiography, and therefore a pigtail catheter will be placed at the origin of the renal arteries for administration of contrast.
3. The bifurcated endograft is evaluated, especially the position of the contralateral limb extracorporeally by fluoroscopy. The main body will be advanced over the Lunderquist wire at the level of the renal arteries. After repeated angiographic scans to identify the exact origin of the lowest renal artery, the endograft is deployed. It is important to minimize the parallax effect of the endograft markers by cranio-caudal movement of the C-arm.
4. The pigtail catheter is removed and the contralateral limb cannulated with a stiff Terumo wire. Alternative catheters for a successful cannulation of the contralateral limb include the Headhunter Shepherd Hook. The next step is testing of the correct position of the pigtail catheter in the endovascular limb of the endoprosthesis. After this, the contralateral limb will be deployed exactly at the iliac bifurcation, preserving the flow to the hypogastric artery.
5. Lastly, the top cap is removed. After deployment of the limb of the bifurcated endograft is completed, a graduated pigtail catheter is advanced and can be helpful to estimate the exact length of the ipsilateral iliac limb. After this step, the iliac limb is deployed just above the iliac bifurcation.

PROCEDURAL ISSUES

Some challenging and technically demanding issues can arise during EVAR.

Challenging Access

Fig. 2.1 illustrates an AAA with severe calcification and stenosis of the iliac arteries and the aortic bifurcation. Several treatment options can be used to overcome this challenging access issue. The first step is to improve the conditions to insert the low-profile endograft by "plain old balloon angioplasty" (POBA). In this case the artery can be predilated with a 7- or 8-mm balloon catheter (Fig. 2.2).

Another option is the "paving and cracking" method. The technique entails the deployment of a balloon-expandable or self-expanding covered stent in the common iliac artery and subsequently, prolonged dilation with a balloon catheter. The benefit is the low risk for

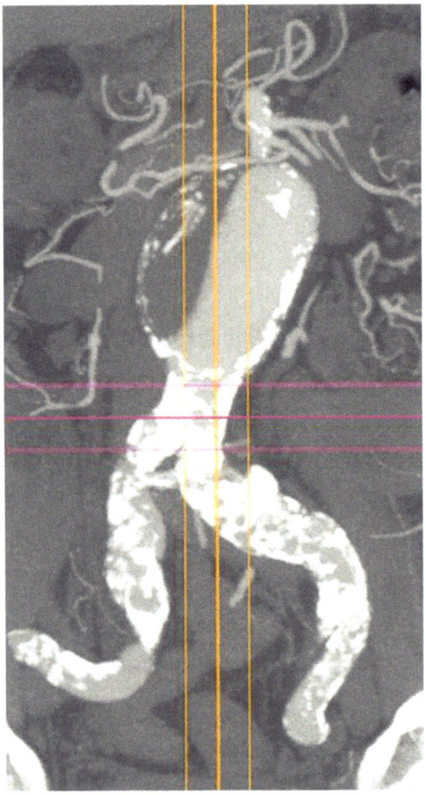

FIG. 2.1 Severe calcification and stenosis of the iliac arteries.

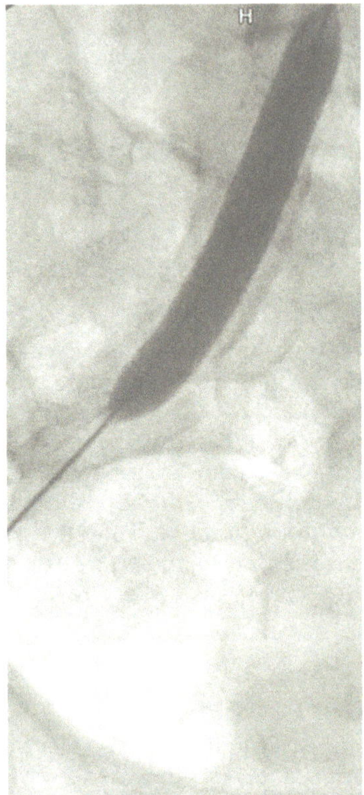

FIG. 2.2 Improving the conditions in EVAR to insert the low-profile endograft by balloon angioplasty, in this case by predilating the artery with a balloon catheter.

iliac hemorrhage from the previously deployed covered stent. A drawback is the possible interaction during the delivery of the endograft with the covered stents, which can lead to migration or fracture of the covered stents. Fig. 2.3 illustrates POBA of the iliac arteries after placement of balloon-expandable covered stents.

The durability of EVAR depends on the maintenance of long-term limb patency. In this context, additional placement of balloon-expandable bare-metal stents at the origin of the iliac limbs is the preferred approach at our Münster center to treat severe stenosis of this segment and small aortic bifurcations with diameter of less than 20 mm. The increase in the radial force of the iliac endovascular limbs by placement of bare-metal stents is crucial to maintain durability of the procedure and long-term patency. Bare-metal stents should be considered whenever a narrow aortic bifurcation or stenosed common iliac arteries are encountered. Fig. 2.4 shows this approach with placement of two balloon-expandable, 10-mm-diameter, 39-mm-long Palmaz stents (Cordis, Baar, Switzerland) in the common iliac arteries.

Another good option for stenosed iliac arteries can be the use of ultralow-profile abdominal endografts such as the INCRAFT endograft (Cordis). Fig. 2.5 illustrates severe bilateral stenoses of the external iliac arteries with luminal diameters of less than 7 mm. The INCRAFT delivery system has an outer diameter (OD) of 14F for all sizes, with exception of the 34 mm, which has an OD of 16F. Fig. 2.6 presents the reconstruction of the successful deployment of the 30-mm INCRAFT device. Our Münster center has 4-year computed tomography angiography (CTA) follow-up with this device showing durability and safety despite the ultralow profile of the endograft.

Challenging Neck: the Angulated Aortic Neck

Deployment of the endograft in a severely angulated aortic neck is challenging. Removal of the tip can also be demanding from interaction with the suprarenal stents. Use of the Endurant device with the short, M-shaped stents can be a good option in this condition (Fig. 2.7).

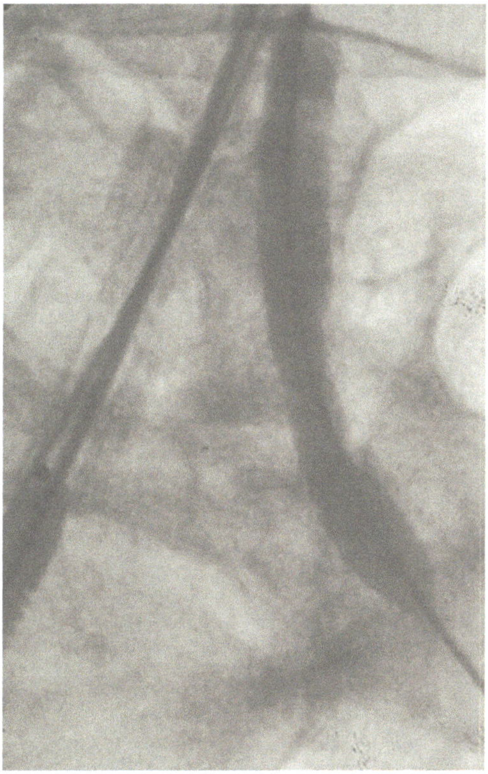

FIG. 2.3 Balloon angioplasty of the iliac arteries after placement of balloon-expandable, covered stents.

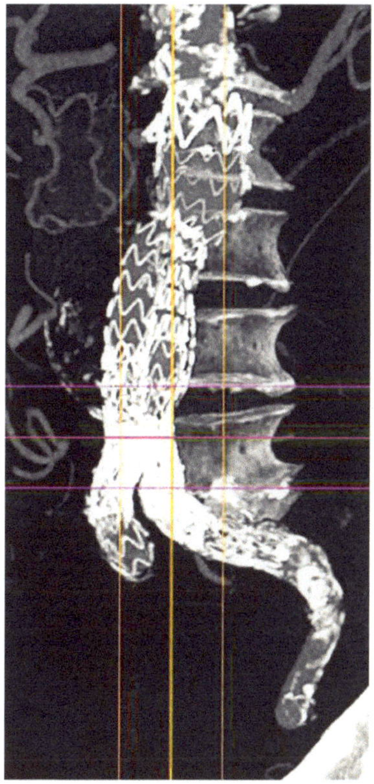

FIG. 2.4 Additional placement of two balloon-expandable stents in the common iliac arteries. This approach improves the radial force of the Endurant limbs in heavily calcified common iliac arteries and minimizes the risk for limb occlusion.

One useful technique to achieve accurate placement is the release of the suprarenal stent and hooks before the full expansion of the proximal segment. This facilitates correction of the position of the endograft without the risk of dissecting the aortic wall, with final deployment of the proximal aspect of the device exactly at the origin of the lowest renal artery.

Severe Pararenal Thrombus Formation

Endografts with infrarenal fixation can be beneficial in cases of severe thrombus formation in the renal or pararenal aortic segment. Fig. 2.8 shows intraoperative angiograms of a challenging case with severe thrombus formation in the pararenal aorta. The patient, who also had an elongated right iliac artery, underwent successful placement of an Excluder C3 (Gore, Tempe, Arizona, USA) bifurcated endograft with infrarenal fixation.

LITERATURE REVIEW

Numerous studies have shown excellent technical success and early outcome with the last-generation stent-grafts. The Endurant stent-graft system was routinely used in our institution as standard abdominal endografts for infrarenal AAAs. The device showed excellent early performance and long-term durability, with few complications or endoleaks requiring reintervention.[3] These satisfactory results were also noted for the patients treated outside the instructions for use (IFU), who were not suitable for treatment by fenestrated endografting because of severe iliac or neck angulation, calcification, and stenosis. The differences between the two subgroups were not statistically significant. Freedom from secondary interventions was 93.3%, 91.6%, and 80.9% at 1, 2, and 5 years, respectively. These results should not lead one to disregard the IFU and perform EVAR indiscriminately in off-label (OL) cases. Nevertheless, when OL conditions are present without other possible options, satisfactory results can be achieved.[4]

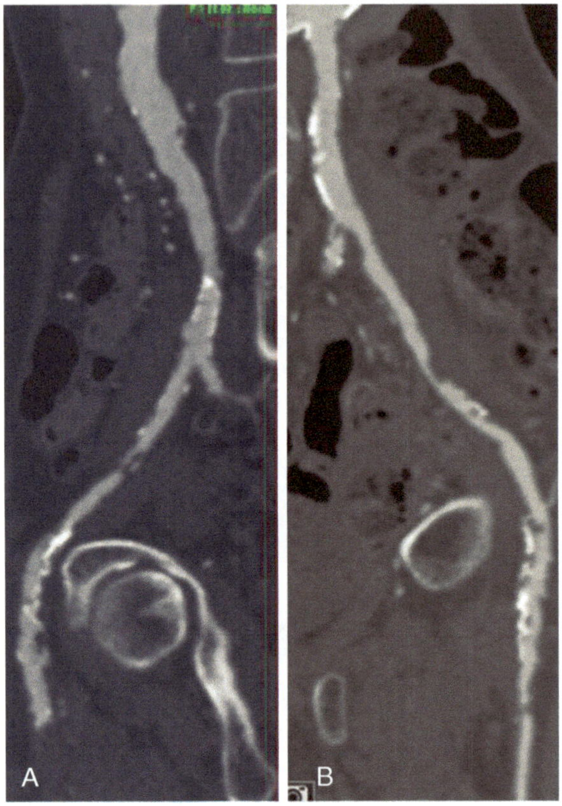

FIG. 2.5 **A, B,** Severe bilateral stenoses of the external iliac arteries with luminal diameters of less than 7 mm.

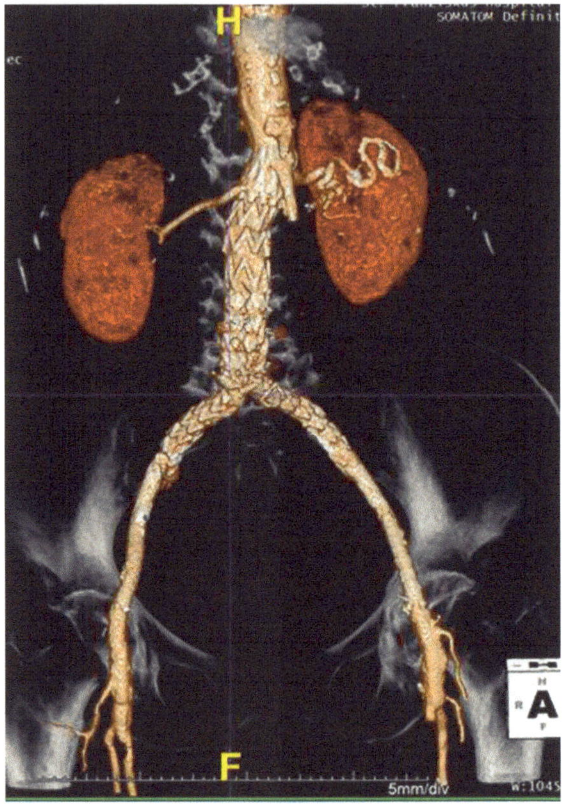

FIG. 2.6 Reconstruction of the successful deployment of the 30-mm INCRAFT device.

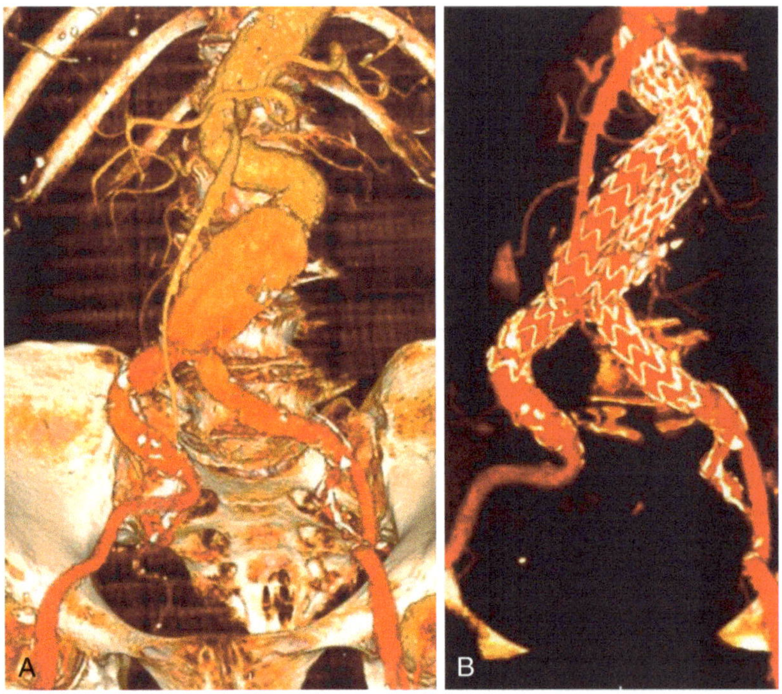

FIG. 2.7 **A, B,** Endurant device with short, M-shaped stents can be used for a severely angulated neck.

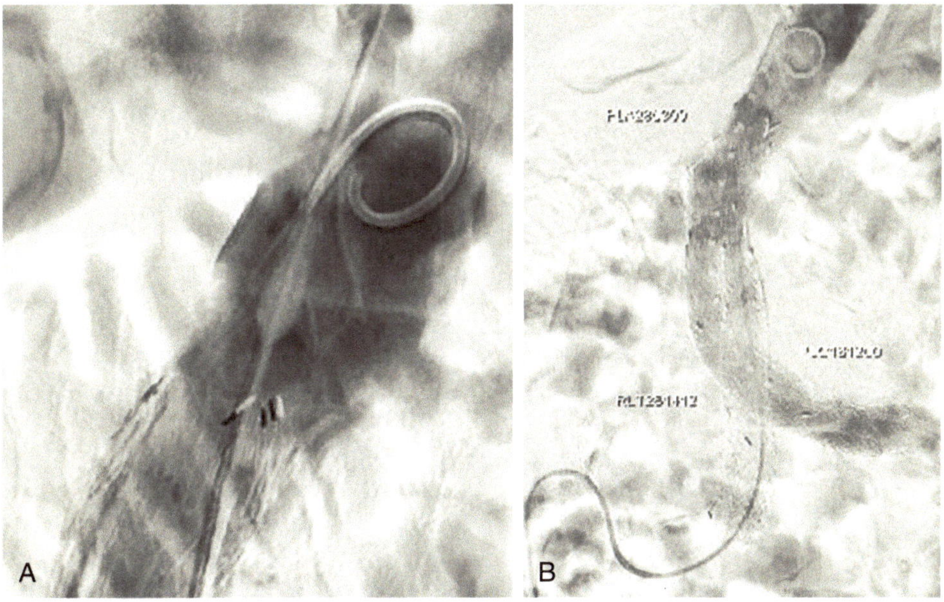

FIG. 2.8 **A, B,** Placement of an Excluder device with infrarenal fixation minimizing the risk of thrombus embolization in the renovisceral vessels in case of thrombus formation at the orifice of the renal arteries.

In 2011, Torsello et al.[5] reported treatment results of 56 patients with Endurant in OL conditions; 27 patients (48.2%) had a proximal aortic neck of less than 10 mm, 22 (39.3%) had infrarenal angulation greater than 75%, and the remaining seven had both anatomic conditions. The 1-year freedom from type I endoleak was 100% in the IFU versus 93.3% in the OL group.

Our center's 2.1% limb occlusion rate with the Endurant device is one of the lowest reported rates in the literature. In 2013 a multicenter Dutch study reported a 4.0% Endurant limb occlusion rate.[6] The main observation of the study was that 90% of the limb occlusions occurred within the first year postoperatively. The authors recommend an aggressive approach with early reintervention to reduce the incidence of occlusion. Our group agrees with this recommendation. A possible explanation for the low incidence of occlusion may be our strategy of deploying additional balloon-expandable bare-metal stents in the common iliac arteries for severe calcification and significant stenosis on the final operative angiogram. In addition, the final angiogram should be always obtained after removal of the stiff wires in order to detect limb misplacement and stenosis, which can lead to early limb occlusion.

REFERENCES

1. Volodos NL, Shekhanin VE, Karpovich IP, et al. A self-fixing synthetic blood vessel endoprosthesis. *Vestn Khir Im II Grek*. 1986;137(11):123–125.
2. Parodi JC, Palmaz JC, Barone HD. Transfemoral intraluminal graft implantation for abdominal aortic aneurysms. *Ann VascSurg*. 1991;5(6):491–499.
3. Donas KP, Torsello G, Weiss K, et al. Performance of the Endurant stent graft in patients with abdominal aortic aneurysms independent of their morphologic suitability for endovascular aneurysm repair based on instructions for use. *J Vasc Surg*. 2015;62(4):848–854.
4. Troisi N, Torsello G, Donas KP, Austermann M. Endurant stent-graft: a 2-year, single-center experience with a new commercially available device for the treatment of abdominal aortic aneurysms. *J Endovasc Ther*. 2010;396: 801–810.
5. Torsello G, Troisi N, Donas KP, Austermann M. Evaluation of the Endurant stent graft under instructions for use vs off-label conditions for endovascular aortic aneurysm repair. *J Vasc Surg*. 2011;54(2):300–306.
6. Van Zeggeren L, Bastos Gonçalves F, van Herwaarden JA, et al. Incidence and treatment results of Endurant endograft occlusion. *J Vasc Surg*. 2013;57(5):1246–1254.

CHAPTER 3

Use of EndoAnchors in Endovascular Treatment of Aneurysms with Short Neck

NICOLA TROISI • EMILIANO CHISCI • STEFANO MICHELAGNOLI • EFTHYMIOS BEROPOULIS

Endovascular aneurysm repair (EVAR) with standard devices can be challenging in cases with "hostile" aortic necks.[1] Several studies have confirmed a close relationship between proximal neck morphology and complications such as type I endoleak. Most authors define a "hostile neck" as one with marked angulation, short length, complex shape, or the presence of calcification or thrombus.[2-4] A challenging aortic neck represents one of the most significant limitations for the endovascular treatment of abdominal aortic aneurysm (AAA).[5-10]

The use of EndoAnchors may be an alternative approach to establish a secure sealing of the endograft during initial EVAR procedures and to treat intraoperative or late type Ia endoleak (Fig. 3.1).[1,11-22]

ENDOANCHOR DEPLOYMENT

The Heli-FX EndoAnchor System (Medtronic Endovascular, Santa Rosa, California, USA) consists of the helical anchors, the EndoAnchor implant (supplied in a cassette containing 10 EndoAnchors), the Heli-FX Applier (a catheter-based device for placement of the EndoAnchor), and the Heli-FX Guide (a deflectable sheath to position the Applier). The system is designed to attach an endograft to the aortic wall by endovascularly placed screws. The EndoAnchors are manufactured from medical-grade nickel-cobalt wire in a helical shape. The leading end is sharpened to a conical point to act as an integral needle, facilitating atraumatic but adequate deployment through the endograft into the vessel wall up to the media, without penetrating the adventitia.

The Heli-FX Applier implants one EndoAnchor at a time using a motorized, two-stage deployment mechanism with reposition ability. It can be used to implant multiple EndoAnchors in a single patient. The Heli-FX Applier is a 12-French (l2F) (outer diameter [OD]) catheter with an integrated control handle.

The Heli-FX Guide is a sterile, single-use, disposable device designed to direct the Heli-FX Applier to the desired location for EndoAnchor implantation. The guide has a high degree of fluoroscopic visibility. The device is compatible with a 0.035-inch guidewire. The Heli-FX Guide consists of a 12F-compatible (inner diameter [ID]) guide sheath with integrated control handle and a matching obturator. Deflection of the distal tip of the catheter is accomplished by rotating the control knob located on the control handle. The Heli-FX Guide is available in both 62-cm (low-profile l6F OD) and 90-cm (l8F OD) working lengths. Multiple deflectable tip lengths are available to accommodate a range of aortic diameters.

INDICATIONS

According to the instructions for use, the Heli-FX EndoAnchor system is intended for use where augmented radial fixation or endograft sealing is required to maintain (prophylactic) or regain (therapeutic) adequate aneurysm exclusion. Furthermore, this system is intended to treat type Ia endoleaks at the initial implantation or in late-onset cases where sealing has been lost because of proximal neck expansion, device deficiencies (e.g., fracture of suprarenal stent supporting structures), or other problems that result in loss of adequate sealing. When loss of seal is accompanied by endograft migration, EndoAnchors must be used in conjunction with aortic extension cuffs to restore sealing to the renal artery level.

INITIAL EXPERIENCE (STAPLE TRIALS)

In a 2009 prospective, single-arm study (STAPLE-1), 21 patients enrolled at five U.S. centers received 96 EndoAnchors (range, 2-10; median, 4).[11] All patients completed 1-month and 6-month follow-up evaluation, and 14

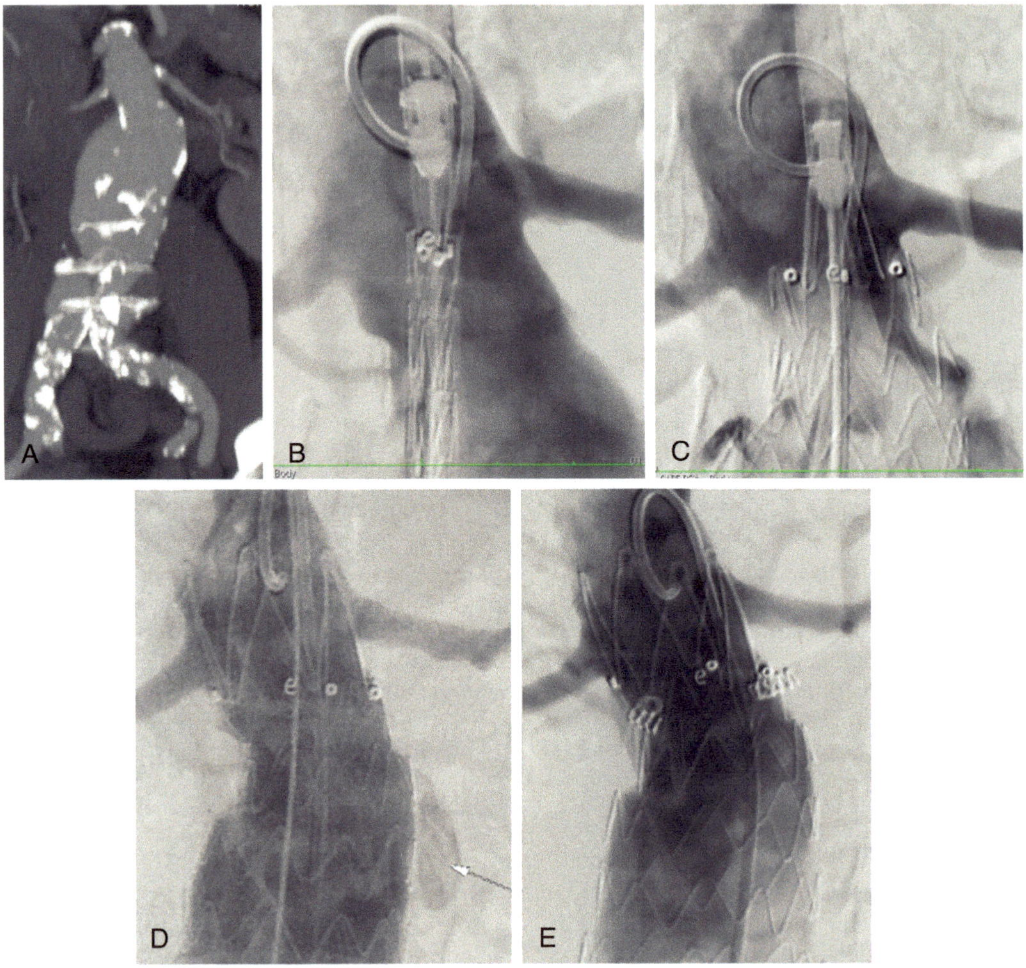

FIG. 3.1 Abdominal aortic aneurysm with hostile proximal aortic neck: **A,** preoperative CT scan; **B,** insertion of endograft; **C,** deployment of the endograft; **D,** detection of type I endoleak; **E,** no endoleak after implantation of Endoanchors.

had 1-year follow-up. Two proximal cuffs were used as adjunctive endograft components at implantation. No further interventions in the proximal aortic neck were performed during the follow-up. Preliminary results of the STAPLE-1 trial demonstrated excellent 6-month and 1-year results.

In 2012, Mehta et al.[12] reported the 24-month outcomes of the STAPLE-2 study of 155 patients; 147 and 121 patients completed 1-year and 2-year follow-up, respectively. A total of 810 EndoAnchors were implanted (median, 5/patient) in conjunction with the Aptus endograft, a device designed without an inherent fixation mechanism, instead relying on EndoAnchors to maintain stability. There were no late type I or III endoleaks. Two cases of migration were observed at the 2-year follow-up, both caused by neck elongation, without actual movement of the endograft from its level of original deployment, and no evidence of graft or staple dislocation, type I endoleak, or reintervention. The authors concluded that the STAPLE-2 trial successfully met the endpoints of safety and efficacy, with aneurysm sac regression in many patients and few reinterventions during the 2-year follow-up. The 3-year outcomes of the STAPLE-2 trial confirmed persistently low rates of type Ia and III endoleaks and reintervention.[13]

ANCHOR TRIAL

The Aneurysm Treatment Using the Heli-FX Aortic Securement System Global Registry (ANCHOR) trial is a multinational registry of EndoAnchor use in a variety of endografts, for prophylaxis against proximal neck problems in patients with hostile aortic neck anatomy, or as therapy when type Ia endoleak or endograft migration occurs. The preliminary 1-month outcomes of the ANCHOR trial reported in 2013 involved 149 patients at 23 U.S. and four European centers over 15 months.[14] The most common indication for EndoAnchor use was a hostile neck in primary procedures (88%) and existing type Ia endoleak in redo procedures (76%). Procedural success was 99% (109 of 110 patients) in primary procedures and 92% (35/38) in redo procedures. Absence of type Ia endoleak was reported in 97% (96/99) and 89% (32/36) of patients, respectively, at 1 month.

In 2014 the early outcomes of the ANCHOR trial were reported.[15] Over a 2-year period, 319 patients were enrolled at 43 sites in the United States and Europe. The study included 242 patients undergoing first-time EVAR (primary arm) and 77 patients with proximal neck complications remote from the initial endograft implantation (revision arm). Over a median imaging follow-up of 7 months, 183 of 202 patients (90.1%) remained free of type Ia endoleaks. The authors concluded that EndoAnchor implantation can be a useful adjunct to EVAR as prophylaxis against proximal attachment site complications in patients with hostile aortic neck anatomy or endograft migration. The most challenging patients, however, presented with type Ia endoleaks remote from initial EVAR; success rates were substantially lower in this group.

Outcomes over longer follow-up were reported in late 2014. Jordan et al.[16] found freedom from secondary procedures in 94.4% of patients (301/319) over mean follow-up of 9.3 months. Among the 18 secondary procedures, eight were performed for residual type Ia endoleaks, and the others were unrelated to EndoAnchors. Use of EndoAnchors to treat existing (late) and acute (at initial endograft implantation) type Ia endoleaks was successful in most cases. Even prophylactic use of EndoAnchors in patients with hostile aortic neck anatomy appeared promising, but robust conclusions must await long-term follow-up data.

The 14-month follow-up outcomes of the ANCHOR trial were reported in 2015. Among 130 of 208 patients with postprocedure computed tomography angiography (CTA), core laboratory analysis identified two patients (1.5%) with persistent type Ia endoleaks. Jordan et al.[17] concluded that prophylactic EndoAnchor use for challenging aortic neck anatomy was associated with satisfactory midterm results.

SINGLE-CENTER EXPERIENCE

Several single-center experiences with EndoAnchors in prophylactic or therapeutic use have been reported. Perdikides et al.[18] investigated the feasibility and early results of endoanchoring as an adjunctive procedure during EVAR in 13 patients with an unfavorable proximal aortic neck. No further proximal aortic neck complications occurred over a median follow-up of 7 months.

Zacharias et al.[19] compared the outcomes of 185 EndoAnchor EVAR patients with 2701 EVAR-only patients. Over mean follow-up of 26 months, EVAR patients had a significantly lower occurrence of nonfatal complications, type Ia endoleak, all types of endoleaks, and need for secondary interventions.

In the first report of EndoAnchor use during an endovascular reintervention, de Vries et al.[20] noted the successful deployment of EndoAnchors in two patients with distally migrated endograft. Hogendoorn et al.[21] reported successful treatment of a ruptured AAA after previous EVAR caused by type Ia endoleak, with deployment of nine EndoAnchors. Chaudhuri[22] reported the successful treatment of a type I endoleak in a patient with a hyperangulated proximal aortic neck.

At Leipzig Interventional Course (LINC) 2017 (Leipzig), Donas presented a 19-patient series of highly selected, multimorbid patients with type Ia endoleaks at the initial EVAR procedure. Other complex endovascular procedures, or open repair, were not feasible in this group. All patients were free from type Ia endoleak, with a statistically significant regression of the aneurysm sac over midterm follow-up.

FUTURE PERSPECTIVES

Despite numerous reports on the outcome of EndoAnchors in EVAR, their ultimate use has not been conclusively demonstrated over long-term follow-up and in the broad spectrum of patients with proximal aortic neck challenges. In a systematic 2013 review, Bail et al.[23] found that the results were not conclusive. Although high-risk patients with unfavorable aneurysm anatomy may benefit from lower reintervention rates after EVAR, randomized controlled trials (RCTs) with larger numbers of patients are needed.

In summary, there is currently a gap in available literature, and the challenge of EndoAnchors is to demonstrate durability over long-term follow-up, assessing the rate of migration or type Ia endoleak and the rate of reinterventions related to proximal aortic neck disease. Moreover, the use of the device to treat intraoperative type Ia endoleak must be further investigated before definitive conclusions on the prophylactic use of EndoAnchors can be formulated.

The indications for EndoAnchors have been expanded to include application in complicated thoracic endovascular aortic procedures,[24] or for repositioning of migrated or malpositioned endografts into the iliac axis (EndoAnchor capture technique).[25-27] Currently, these applications have been reported anecdotally, and the value of such applications remains to be evaluated with more robust data.

REFERENCES

1. Jordan Jr WD, Ouriel K, Mehta M, et al. Aneurysm Treatment using the Heli-FX Aortic Securement System Global Registry ANCHOR. Outcome-based anatomic criteria for defining the hostile aortic neck. *J Vasc Surg*. 2015;61:1383–1390.
2. Buckley CJ, Buckley SD. Limitations of current EVAR endografts and potential solutions for their deficiencies. *Semin Vasc Surg*. 2012;25:136–137.
3. Buckley CJ, Buckley SD. Deficiencies with current aortic endografts. *J Cardiovasc Surg*. 2015;56:369–373.
4. Navarro TP, Bernardes Rde C, Procopio RJ, Leite JO, Dardik A. Treatment of hostile proximal necks during endovascular aneurysm repair. *Aorta*. 2014;2:28–36.
5. De Vries JP. The proximal neck: the remaining barrier to a complete EVAR world. *Semin Vasc Surg*. 2012;25:182–186.
6. Troisi N, Torsello G. New-generation devices and adjunctive procedures are the key elements to expanding the indications for endovascular aneurysm repair. *J Endovasc Ther*. 2015;22:179–181.
7. Donas KP, Lee JT, Lachat M, Torsello G, Veith FJ; PERICLES investigators. Collected world experience about the performance of the snorkel/chimney endovascular technique in the treatment of complex aortic pathologies: the PERICLES registry. Ann Surg 201;262:546-553; discussion 552–553.
8. Pecoraro F, Veith FJ, Puippe G, et al. Mid- and longer-term follow up of chimney and/or periscope grafts and risk factors for failure. *Eur J Vasc Endovasc Surg*. 2016;51:664–673.
9. Chisci E, Ventoruzzo G, Alamanni N, Bellandi G, Michelagnoli S. Transrenal E-XL stenting to resolve or prevent type Ia endoleak in the case of severe neck angulation during endovascular abdominal aortic aneurysm repair. *J Vasc Surg*. 2013;57:1383–1386.
10. Deaton DH. Improving proximal fixation and seal with the Heli-Fx aortic EndoAnchor. *Semin Vasc Surg*. 2012;25:187–192.
11. Deaton DH, Mehta M, Kasirajan K, et al. The phase I multicenter trial (STAPLE-1) of the Aptus endovascular repair system: results at 6 months and 1 year. *J Vasc Surg*. 2009;49:851–857; discussion 857–858.
12. Mehta M, Fairman RM, Deaton DH. Staple-2: the pivotal study of the Aptus endovascular AAA repair system—24-months results. *J Vasc Surg*. 2012;55:624.
13. Mehta M, Henretta J, Glickman M, et al. Outcome of the pivotal study of the Aptus endovascular abdominal aortic aneurysms repair system. *J Vasc Surg*. 2014;60:275–285.
14. Jordan Jr WD, de Vries JP, Mehta M, Varnagy D, Joye J. Prospective multicenter international trial of EndoAnchor fixation and sealing of aortic endografts: indications for use and early results in the ANCHOR trial. *J Vasc Surg*. 2013;58:857.
15. De Vries JP, Ouriel K, Mehta M, et al. Aneurysm Treatment Using the Heli-FX Aortic Securement System Global Registry ANCHOR Trial. Analysis of EndoAnchors for endovascular aneurysm repair by indications for use. *J Vasc Surg*. 2014;60:1460–1467.
16. Jordan Jr WD, Mehta M, Varnagy D, et al. Results of the ANCHOR prospective, multicenter registry of EndoAnchors for type Ia endoleaks and endograft migration in patients with challenging anatomy. *J Vasc Surg*. 2014;60:885–892.
17. Jordan Jr WD, de Vries JP, Ouriel K, et al. Midterm outcome of EndoAnchors for the prevention of endoleak and stent-graft migration in patients with challenging proximal aortic neck anatomy. *J Endovasc Ther*. 2015;22:163–170.
18. Perdikides T, Melas N, Lagios K, et al. Primary endoanchoring in the endovascular repair of abdominal aortic aneurysms with an unfavorable neck. *J Endovasc Ther*. 2012;19:707–715.
19. Zacharias N, Mehta M, Paty PS, Ouriel K. Use of Heli-Fx EndoAnchor during EVAR reduces endoleaks and the need for secondary interventions: a prospective single-center analysis. *J Vasc Surg*. 2015;62:797.
20. De Vries JP, Schrijver AM, Van den Heuvel DA, Vos JA. Use of endostaples to secure migrated endografts and proximal cuffs after failed endovascular abdominal aortic aneurysm repair. *J Vasc Surg*. 2011;54:1792–1794.
21. Hogendoorn W, Schlösser FJ, Aruny JE, Indes JE, Sumpio BE, Muhs BE. Successful treatment of a proximal type I endoleak with Heli-FX EndoAnchors. *Ann Vasc Surg*. 2014;28:737.e13-e17.
22. Chaudhuri A. Endostapling can constrain a hyperangulated neck and successfully treat a proximal type I endoleak after EVAR. *Eur J Vasc Endovasc Surg*. 2016;51:681.
23. Bail DH, Walker T, Giehl J. Vascular endostapling systems for vascular endografts (T)EVAR: systematic review—current state. *Vasc Endovascular Surg*. 2013;47:261–266.
24. Ongstad SB, Miller DF, Panneton JM. The use of EndoAnchors to rescue complicated TEVAR procedures. *J Cardiovasc Surg*. 2016;57:716–729.
25. Garland BT, Singh N, Starnes BW. Endovascular repositioning of a migrated stent graft using "endoanchor capture". *Ann Vasc Surg*. 2015;29:123.e1-e5.
26. Katsargyris A, Oikonomou K, Klonaris C. Comparison of outcomes with open, fenestrated, and chimney graft repair of juxtarenal aneurysms: are we ready for a paradigm shift? *J Endovasc Ther*. 2013;20(2):159–169.
27. Melas N, Perdikides T, Saratzis A, et al. A novel approach to minimize sealing defects: EndoAnchors reduce gutter size in an in vitro chimney graft model. *J Endovasc Ther*. 2013;20:506–513.

CHAPTER 4

Use of Contrast-Enhanced Ultrasound in Follow-up of Endovascular Aneurysm Repair

EMILIANO CHISCI • NICOLA TROISI • STEFANO MICHELAGNOLI

The optimal protocol for imaging and timing of endovascular aortic aneurysm repair (EVAR) follow-up is still being developed. Various follow-up modalities are employed to measure aortic sac diameter, to detect and classify endoleaks, to detect morphologic details of the stent-graft (e.g., graft occlusion), and to detect imaging evidence of endograft infection and other details.[1,2] A recent systematic review reported that more than 90% of EVAR patients undergoing follow-up do not benefit from surveillance, since imaging alone initiates asymptomatic secondary interventions (SIR) in only 1.4% to 9% of patients.[3-6] Therefore the least invasive and safest EVAR follow-up protocol is needed so that radiation-induced and other complications from surveillance imaging do not exceed the risk of complications from EVAR itself. The "Achilles' heel" of EVAR is the presence of endoleak and the indication/timing for SIR, especially for type II endoleaks, the most commonly encountered variety. This chapter examines the role of contrast-enhanced ultrasound (CEUS) in the follow-up of patients after EVAR.

LITERATURE REVIEW

A real-time imaging modality, CEUS is gaining popularity in different settings of vascular medicine because it has zero potential morbidity and no risk of contrast-induced nephropathy or radiation exposure. This is in marked contrast to the current "gold standard" technique of computed tomography angiography (CTA). CEUS has emerged as an additional modality to enhance color duplex ultrasound, with the potential to better detect and classify the type of endoleak and target-vessel patency. CEUS allows for superior visualization of the aorta and its main branches. CEUS is the result of synergic integration between ultrasound contrast agents and dedicated hardware and software platforms. The endograft can be visualized with CEUS over approximately 5 to 10 minutes, imaging the endograft from different angles to assess the perfused lumen and evaluate low-flow states with high temporal resolution. Thrombotic material can be appreciated as a focal filling defect, located at the wall of the aneurysm sac or adjacent to the endograft.

The agents used in CEUS are stabilized microspheres consisting of sulfur hexafluoride or perfluorocarbon encapsulated by a phospholipid shell. Ultrasound contrast agents are administered by intravenous injection and are strictly confined in the vascular space (blood-pool agents), where they strongly enhance the blood's acoustic signal. Ultrasound microbubbles act similar to red blood cells. The effectiveness of these contrast agents depends on their echogenicity (ability of gas inside microbubbles to reflect ultrasound), concentration (number of bubbles), and harmonic answer (special behavior of bubbles when exposed to ultrasound beam). These microbubbles show nonlinear behavior when examined on an ultrasound machine with a low mechanical index.

Reports show that CEUS has high sensitivity and specificity in detecting endoleaks compared with CTA, with values of 92% to 100% and 82% to 100%, respectively.[7-17] CEUS imaging has proved to be as good as CTA in detecting endoleaks because of its real-time dynamic nature. It is even better able to quantify flow and characterize the different endoleak types than CTA because of the latter's limited ability to show the direction of flow. CEUS can be as sensitive as CTA in detecting the endoleaks that would normally warrant an immediate intervention (types I and III), as well as endoleaks (type II) that CTA might miss. CEUS can help determine the origin of these endoleaks and can provide ultrasound parameters of type II endoleaks that predict a high risk for aneurysm sac pressurization and rupture.

High-flow endoleaks are detected with simultaneous enhancement inside and outside the graft in types I and III (Figs. 4.1 and 4.2). For type II endoleaks, the source of the nidus can be identified (Fig. 4.3). With

Type I Endoleak

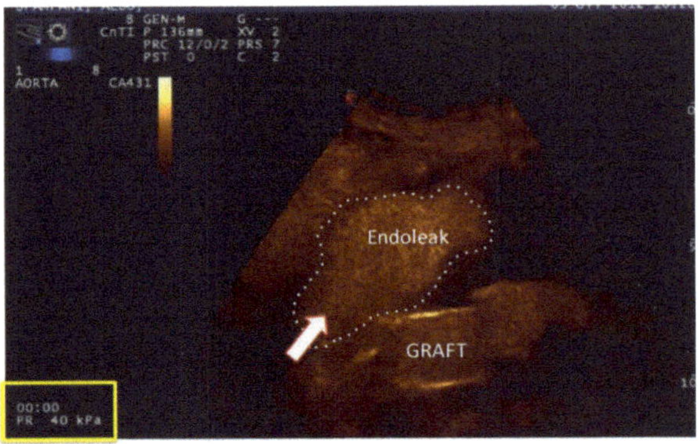

FIG. 4.1 High-flow type I endoleak with simultaneous enhancement inside and outside the graft (time 0 second). Contrast-enhanced ultrasound (CEUS) was performed with a bolus of 5 mL Sonovue.

type IV endoleaks, however, no enhancement outside the graft is detectable, even in very late phase (>2 minutes) (Fig. 4.4). An important role for CEUS is the follow-up of patients with previous EVAR who received SIR with coils, plugs, or glues. In this setting, CEUS is reliable for monitoring coil-embolized sacs containing tantalum-enhanced glues, avoiding artifacts inherent in CTA images. Moreover, Gargiulo et al.[18] suggested the use of three-dimensional (3D) CEUS for follow-up of fenestrated EVAR, providing a reconstruction of the fenestrated endograft and its target vessels that is easier to interpret than CTA or two-dimensional (2D) CEUS.

Since 2011, the European Federation of Societies for Ultrasound in Medicine and Biology has recommended CEUS for the detection, classification, and follow-up of abdominal aortic aneurysm (AAA) endoleaks.[19] CEUS has some limitations as the sole imaging modality for EVAR surveillance, however, because of its "operator dependency" and certain patient characteristics, such as obesity (body mass index [BMI] >30), ascites, and conditions with abundant intestinal gas, which can create technical problems. Another potential disadvantage of CEUS is its relative inability to detect fractures or component separation of the metal skeleton of an endograft.

San Giovanni di Dio Hospital Experience

The CEUS experience at the San Giovanni di Dio Hospital, Florence, Italy, is one of the largest for EVAR follow-up.[20,21] We have performed CEUS routinely for EVAR follow-up since 1999, when the first EVAR procedure was performed at our center.

At the beginning, EVAR surveillance at our tertiary referral center was based on plain abdominal radiography (RX), color duplex ultrasound (CDU), and CTA. From 2012, CEUS was performed for the following indications:

- Detection of an endoleak
- Significant aneurysm expansion (e.g., sac growth >5 mm within 6 months)
- Patient with renal insufficiency (e.g., ≥stage 3 chronic kidney disease [CKD] classification)
- Patient with iodine contrast allergy

Our current postoperative EVAR protocol is a 1-month follow-up consisting of CTA, CDU, plain RX, and clinical checkup. CEUS is performed selectively, based on the four indications. Thereafter, clinical checkup, CDU, and plain RX are performed every 6 months. Currently, CTA is reserved in our center for any abnormalities or nondiagnostic imaging, or to plan SIR.

A standard CDU is always performed before CEUS. After overnight fasting, a sagittal or transverse scan of the supine patient is performed using the probe. B-mode imaging is used initially to identify the aorta, while the maximum diameter of the aneurysmal sac is measured in the transverse plane. The patency of renal arteries is confirmed using spectral Doppler ultrasound. The aorta is scanned from the proximal attachment site of the endograft to the distal point. Using color and spectral Doppler ultrasound, the stent is assessed for perigraft flow, graft stenosis, thrombosis, kinking, and endoleaks, according to the reporting standards for EVAR.[2]

CEUS is then performed with the same ultrasound machine; always by an experienced vascular surgeon. A low mechanical index (varying from 0.2 to 0.30) is used to avoid early destruction of the microbubbles. A 2.5- to 5-MHz probe (Esaote, Genoa, Italy) is employed. The contrast used is a second-generation agent (SonoVue; Bracco, Milan, Italy) made of sulfur hexafluoride–filled microbubbles with flexible lipid shells, eliminated through the respiratory system. Its use is contraindicated in patients with unstable angina, recent episode of acute coronary syndrome (<14 days), or severe chronic obstructive lung disease with a recent exacerbation. As such, all patients are screened for the contraindications before contrast administration.

Contrast techniques apply a low acoustic pressure to produce images based on nonlinear acoustic interaction between the ultrasound system and the microbubbles. The microbubbles oscillate and resound, allowing continuous display of contrast enhancement

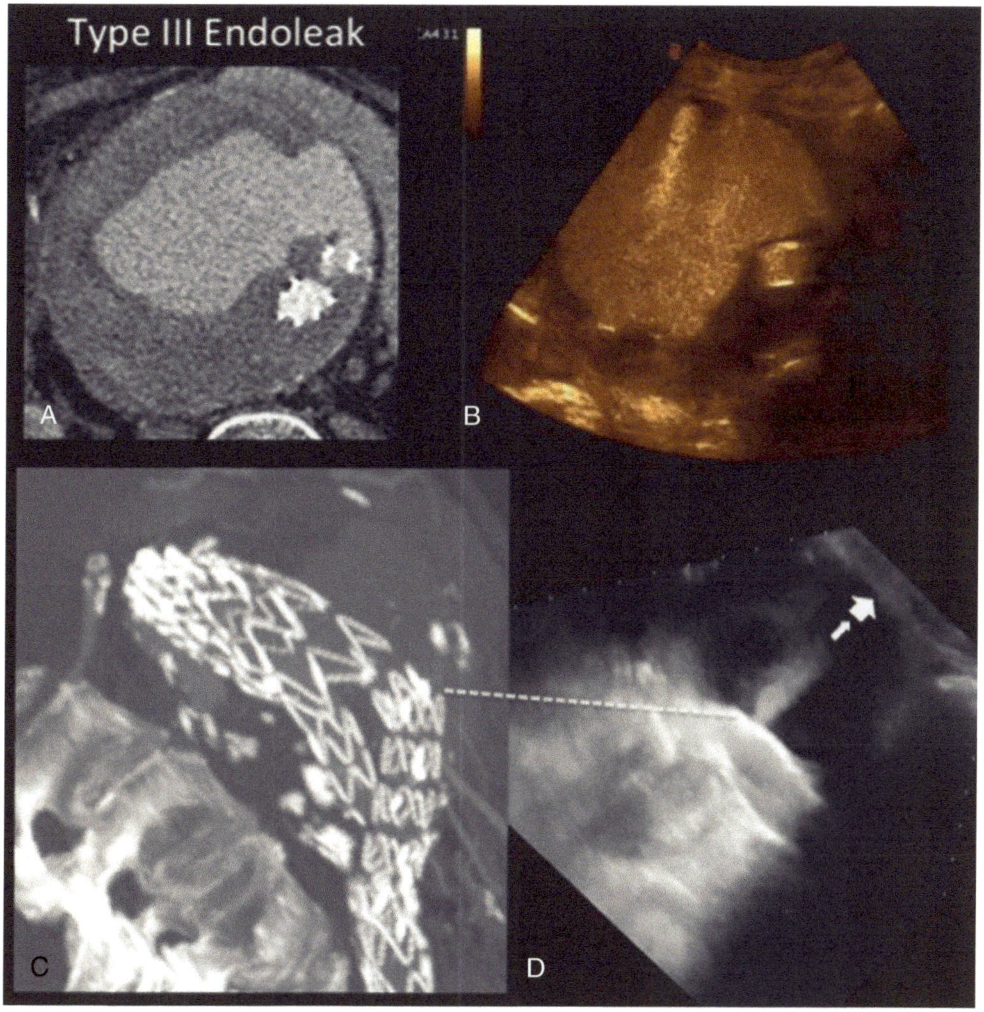

FIG. 4.2 High-flow type III endoleaks at **A,** computed tomography angiography (CTA), compared with **B,** CEUS (time 2 seconds). CEUS was performed with a bolus of 5 mL Sonovue. **C,** CTA 3D reconstruction demonstrating the proximal limb disconnection from the main body. **D,** B-mode image with contrast agent showing the jet flow from the disconnected graft.

on gray-scale images. A single bolus of 5 mL is administered through an 18-gauge cannula placed in the antecubital fossa, followed by 5 mL of normal saline flush. We prefer to inject this larger amount of contrast agent to increase both sensitivity and specificity of the examination in detecting endoleaks; literature reports a dose of 1 to 2.5 mL for the first bolus, generally with a similar amount of contrast for the second bolus. Immediate endoleak enhancement would suggest a graft-related type I or III endoleak, whereas a delay of greater than 5 seconds suggests a type II endoleak. Indeed, in all patients in this study in whom a type I endoleak was observed, contrast enhancement was seen arriving in the aneurysm and stent-graft simultaneously (see Fig. 4.1).

Findings are reviewed and discussed at a multidisciplinary team meeting of vascular radiologists and vascular surgeons, to arrive at a diagnosis and formulate an appropriate management plan.

Between 2012 and 2016, EVAR surveillance prompted 318 CEUS scans (median age, 78; range, 67-92; 255 males). The main indications for CEUS were the presence of any endoleak (n = 160; 50%); significant aneurysm expansion, with sac growth greater than 5 mm within 6 months

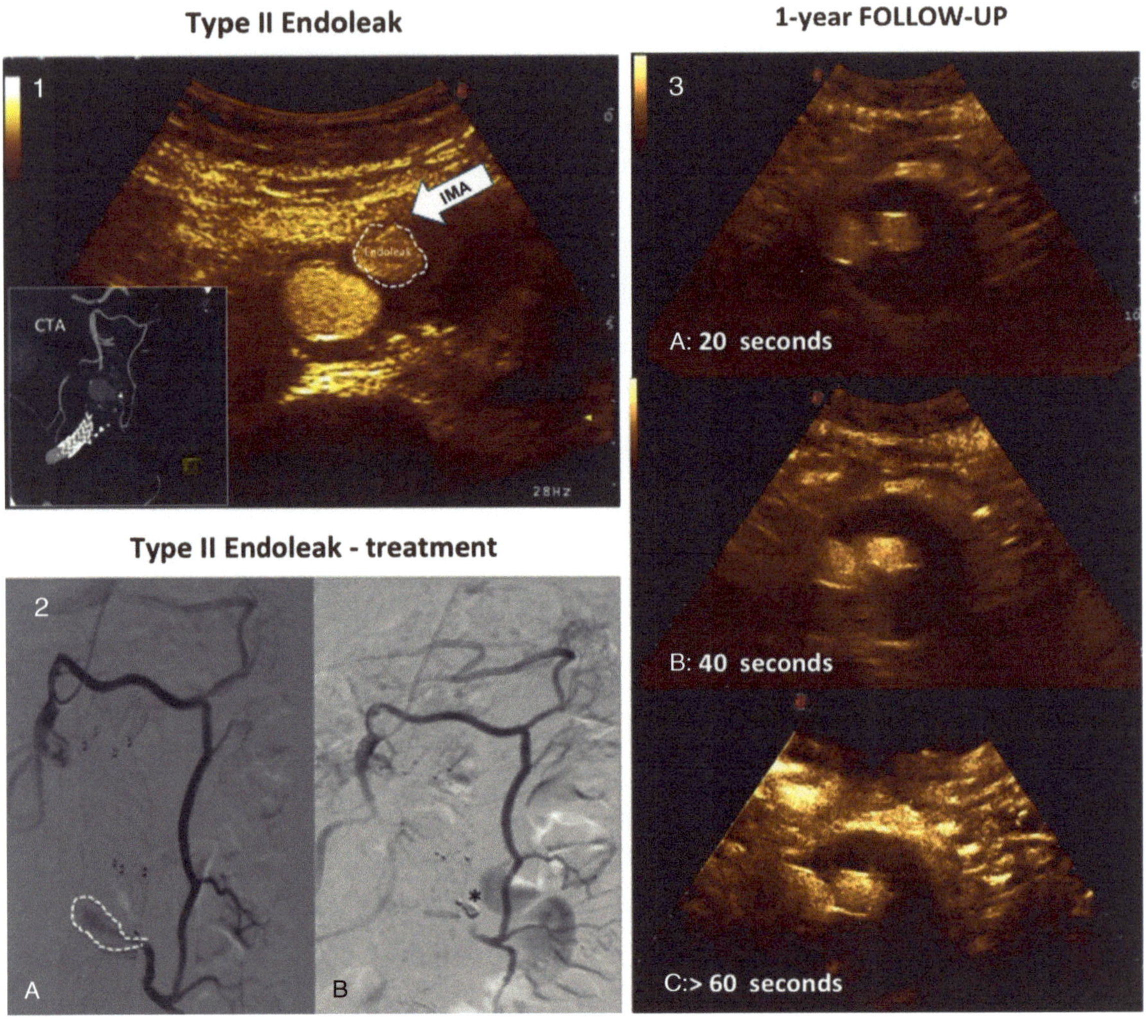

FIG. 4.3 **1,** Low-flow type II endoleak originating from the inferior mesenteric artery (*IMA*). CEUS was performed with a bolus of 5 mL Sonovue (time 20 seconds). Endoleak nidus is highlighted. CTA showing the origin of the type II endoleak from Riolan's arcade. **2, A,** Angiography 4F catheter in superior mesenteric artery + 2.7 microcatheter superselective advancement to IMA origin showing type II endoleaks. **B,** Angiography demonstrating exclusion of endoleaks and patency of intestinal vascularization following coil embolization of IMA origin with 5 × 10 cm detachable coil (×2). **3,** One-year CEUS follow-up demonstrating at 20, 40, and >60 seconds the absence of contrast enhancement of the aneurysmal sac. CEUS was performed with a bolus of 5 mL Sonovue.

(n = 34; 11%); and patients with renal insufficiency (≥stage 3 CKD: n = 91; 29%) or iodine contrast allergy (n = 33; 10%) (Fig. 4.5). Median follow-up after EVAR was 78 months (range, 0-207 months). CEUS was compared to CTA in the first 100 patients and had 100% sensitivity and 100% specificity for classification of endoleaks. Moreover, CTA misclassified two type II endoleaks (one as type I and one as type III). In all cases, CEUS was able to detect and classify endoleaks. The frequency of type I, II, III, and IV endoleaks was 16 (10%), 139 (86%), 3 (2%), and 3 (2%), respectively (Table 4.1). During the 4-year period since CEUS introduction, the rate of SIR for screened patients was 11% (36). Need for SIR was prompted by CEUS when all the following three criteria occurred:

1. Sac growth greater than 5 mm within 6 months
2. Presence of any endoleak

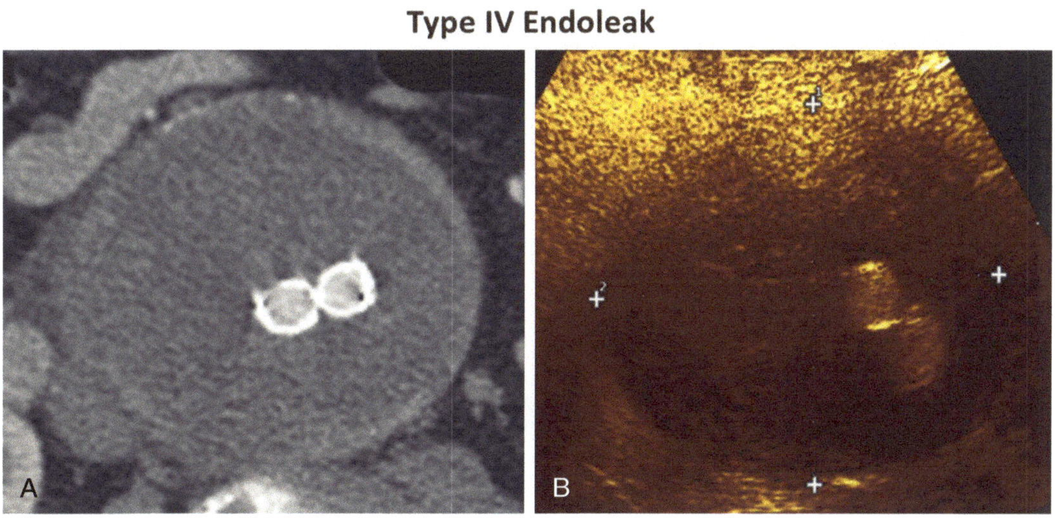

FIG. 4.4 Type IV endoleaks with no-enhancement at **A,** CTA, and **B,** CEUS (>180 seconds). CEUS was performed with a bolus of 5 mL Sonovue.

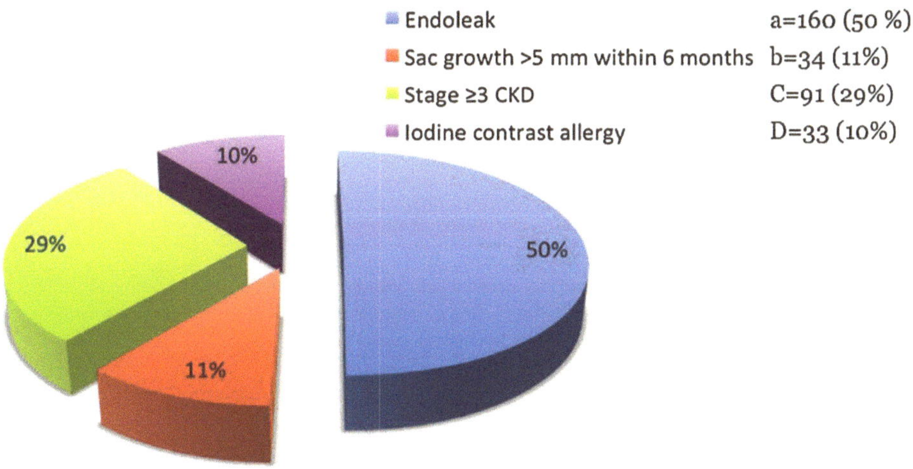

FIG. 4.5 Primary indications for CEUS. *CKD,* Chronic kidney disease.

TABLE 4.1
Type of Endoleak Screened by CEUS Examination

Endoleak Type	*n* (%)	SIR, *n* (%)
Overall	160 (100)	36 (100)
I	18 (10)	15 (42)
II	139 (86)	17 (47)
III	3 (2)	3 (8)
IV	3 (2)	1 (3)

SIR, Secondary interventions.

3. Contrast enhancement persisting longer than 60 seconds

CTA was required before any SIR. Patients not meeting the criteria continued with 6-month standard surveillance (CDU + RX) in 65% of cases (206), including a subsequent CEUS in 24% (76) (Fig. 4.6).

Two aneurysm-related deaths occurred during follow-up; one patient died 6 days before scheduled SIR, and one from cardiac complications of SIR; in both the primary cause of death was the rupture of the aneurysmal sac. CEUS is not less expensive than CTA (currently 120 vs. 125 euros) but has almost no morbidity and

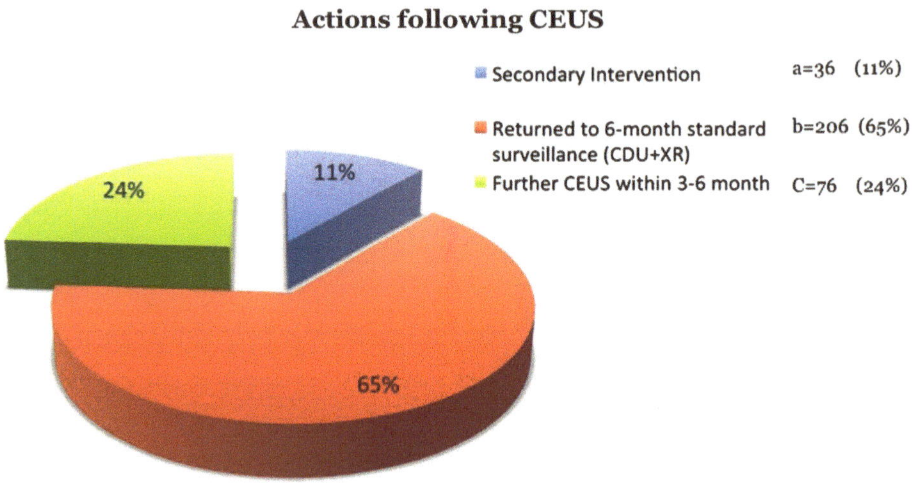

FIG. 4.6 Intervention and EVAR surveillance after CEUS. *CDU,* Color duplex ultrasonography; *RX,* plain abdominal radiography.

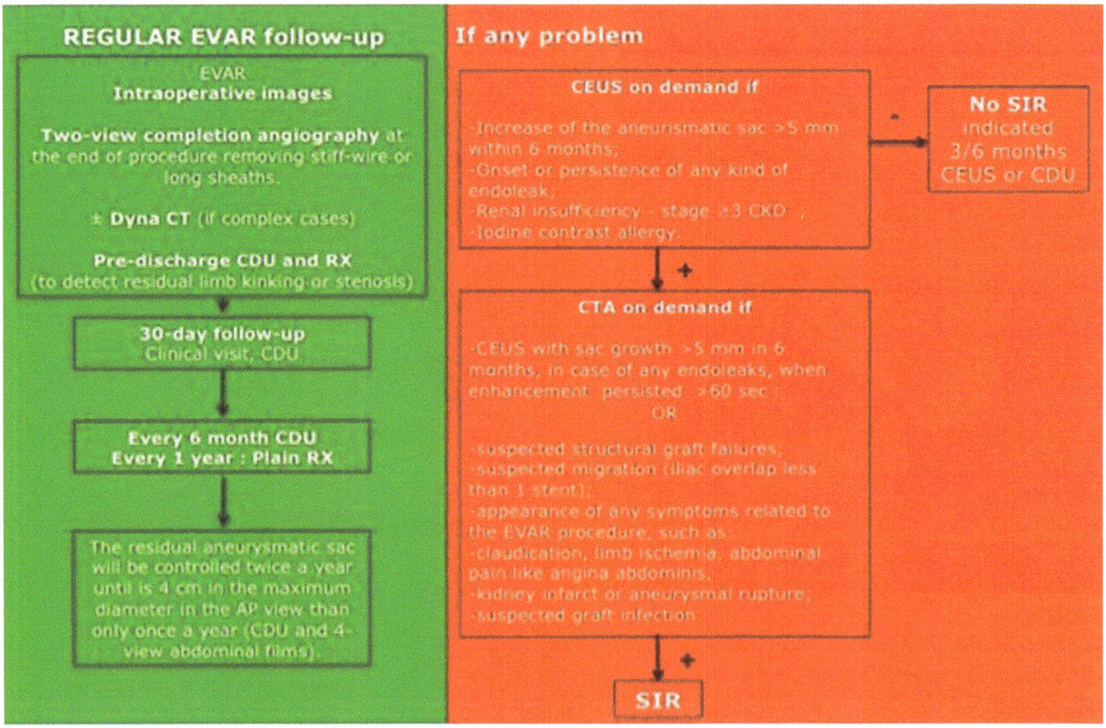

FIG. 4.7 Proposed protocol of surveillance as currently performed in our center. *CDU,* Color duplex ultrasonography; *CKD,* chronic kidney disease; *CTA,* computed tomography angiography; *EVAR,* endovascular aortic aneurysm repair; *RX,* plain abdominal radiography; *SIR,* secondary interventions.

no risk of contrast nephropathy or radiation exposure compared with CTA. We observed no contrast-related complications; patients with allergies were pretreated with cortisone and antihistamines. The advantages of CEUS should be balanced against its cost. A 4-year analysis of CTA use documented a 90% reduction after the introduction of CEUS. Fig. 4.7 shows our current surveillance protocol.

SUMMARY

Contrast-enhanced ultrasound correctly identifies and classifies endoleaks after EVAR. Further, CEUS can accurately guide the need for secondary interventions, using three CEUS criteria (sac growth >5 mm within 6 months, presence of endoleak, contrast enhancement persisting >60 seconds). However, CTA is always necessary to plan a secondary intervention. Data suggest that the use of CEUS can simplify EVAR surveillance, adopting CDU as the main follow-up modality, and performing CEUS and CTA as required in select patients. Surveillance protocols often require a combination of modalities to ensure safe, economically sustainable, and effective EVAR follow-up.

ACKNOWLEDGMENT

We would like to express our deepest appreciation to Ms. Angelica Pecchioli, who has helped us to coordinate the entire EVAR follow-up since 1999, and who embraced with the same enthusiasm and passion the CEUS project at our Vascular Unit.

REFERENCES

1. Moll FL, Powell JT, Fraedrich G, et al. Management of abdominal aortic aneurysms: clinical practice guidelines of the European Society for Vascular Surgery. *Eur J Vasc Endovasc Surg*. 2011;41(suppl 1):S1–S58.
2. Chaikof EL, Brewster DC, Dalman RL, et al. The care of patients with an abdominal aortic aneurysm: the Society for Vascular Surgery practice guidelines. *J Vasc Surg*. 2009;50:S2–49.
3. Nordon IM, Karthikesalingam A, Hinchliffe RJ, et al. Secondary interventions following endovascular aneurysm repair (EVAR) and the enduring value of graft surveillance. *Eur J Vasc Endovasc Surg*. 2010;39:547–554.
4. Dias NV, Riva L, Ivancev K, et al. Is there a benefit of frequent CT follow-up after EVAR? *Eur J Vasc Endovasc Surg*. 2009;37:425–430.
5. Black SA, Carrell TW, Bell RE, et al. Long-term surveillance with computed tomography after endovascular aneurysm repair may not be justified. *Br J Surg*. 2009;96:1280–1283.
6. Chisci E, Setacci F, Iacoponi F, et al. Surveillance imaging modality does not affect detection rate of asymptomatic secondary interventions following EVAR. *Eur J Vasc Endovasc Surg*. 2012;43:276–281.
7. Partovi S, Kaspar M, Aschwanden M, et al. Contrast-enhanced ultrasound after endovascular aortic repair: current status and future perspectives. *Cardiovasc Diagn Ther*. 2015;5:454–463.
8. Bredahl KK, Taudorf M, Lönn L, et al. Contrast-enhanced ultrasound can replace computed tomography angiography for surveillance after endovascular aortic aneurysm repair. *Eur J Vasc Endovasc Surg*. 2016;52:729–734.
9. Abbas A, Hansrani V, Sedgwick N, et al. 3D contrast enhanced ultrasound for detecting endoleak following endovascular aneurysm repair (EVAR). *Eur J Vasc Endovasc Surg*. 2014;47:487–492.
10. Gilabert R, Buñesch L, Real MI, et al. Evaluation of abdominal aortic aneurysm after endovascular repair: prospective validation of contrast-enhanced US with a second-generation US contrast agent. *Radiology*. 2012;264:269–277.
11. Motta R, Rubaltelli L, Vezzaro R, et al. Role of multidetector CT angiography and contrast-enhanced ultrasound in redefining follow-up protocols after endovascular abdominal aortic aneurysm repair. *Radiol Med*. 2012;117:1079–1092.
12. Gürtler VM, Sommer WH, Meimarakis G, et al. A comparison between contrast-enhanced ultrasound imaging and multislice computed tomography in detecting and classifying endoleaks in the follow-up after endovascular aneurysm repair. *J Vasc Surg*. 2013;58:340–345.
13. Iezzi R, Basilico R, Giancristofaro D, et al. Contrast enhanced ultrasound versus color duplex ultrasound imaging in the follow-up of patients after endovascular abdominal aortic aneurysm repair. *J Vasc Surg*. 2009;49:552–560.
14. Chung J, Kordzadeh A, Prionidis I, et al. Contrast-enhanced ultrasound (CEUS) versus computed tomography angiography (CTA) in detection of endoleaks in post-EVAR patients. Are delayed type II endoleaks being missed? A systematic review and meta-analysis. *J Ultrasound*. 2015;18:91–99.
15. Karthikesalingam W, Al-Jundi, Jackson D, et al. Systematic review and meta-analysis of duplex ultrasonography, contrast-enhanced ultrasonography or computed tomography for surveillance after endovascular aneurysm repair. *Br J Surg*. 2012;99:1514–1523.
16. Mirza TA, Karthikesalingam A, Jackson D, et al. Duplex ultrasound and contrast-enhanced ultrasound versus computed tomography for the detection of endoleak after EVAR: systematic review and bivariate meta-analysis. *Eur J Vasc Endovasc Surg*. 2010;39:418–422.
17. Cantisani V, Ricci P, Grazhdani H, Napoli A, Fanelli F, Catalano C. Prospective comparative analysis of colour-Doppler ultrasound, contrast-enhanced ultrasound, computed tomography and magnetic resonance in detecting endoleak after endovascular abdominal aortic aneurysm repair. *Eur J Vasc Endovasc Surg*. 2011;41:186–192.
18. Gargiulo M, Gallitto E, Serra C, et al. Could four-dimensional contrast-enhanced ultrasound replace computed tomography angiography during follow up of fenestrated endografts? Results of a preliminary experience. *Eur J Vasc Endovasc Surg*. 2014;48:536–542.
19. Piscaglia F, Nolsøe C, Dietrich CF, et al. The EFSUMB guidelines and recommendations on the clinical practice of contrast enhanced ultrasound (CEUS): update 2011 on non-hepatic applications. *Ultraschall Med*. 2012;33:33–59.
20. Chisci E, Pigozzi C, Pecchioli A, et al. The role of contrast-enhanced ultrasound in endoleaks surveillance is to define the need of a secondary intervention. *J Vasc Surg*. 2015;61:199S–200S.
21. Chisci E, Pecchioli A, Barbanti E, et al. Three criteria derived from contrast-enhanced ultrasound define when a secondary intervention is needed during endoleaks surveillance. *J Vasc Surg*. 2016;63:82S.

CHAPTER 5

Logistics in the Hybrid Operating Room for Complex Endovascular Aneurysm Repair

KONSTANTINOS P. DONAS • FRANCISCO MARQUES DE AZEVEDO

Endovascular treatment of complex aortic disease requires advanced imaging. The ideal facilities to perform complex endovascular aneurysm repair (EVAR) are the *hybrid* rooms, defined as the synthesis of a fully equipped operating room (OR) with all the necessary diagnostic equipment. Fig. 5.1 shows the first hybrid OR in Germany. This angiosuite was built in 2003 in Münster, at St. Franziskus Hospital for the Department of Vascular Surgery. The hybrid room allows high-quality diagnostic imaging, endovascular interventions, and the option for open surgery. Important characteristics of the angiography system are continuous and pulsed fluoroscopy recording the vascular route and masking overlay, single and sequential shooting power with variable frame rates, four different operating positions of the C-arm, and several programs for radiation exposure protection. The C-arm can be positioned from the console at the table (Fig. 5.2).

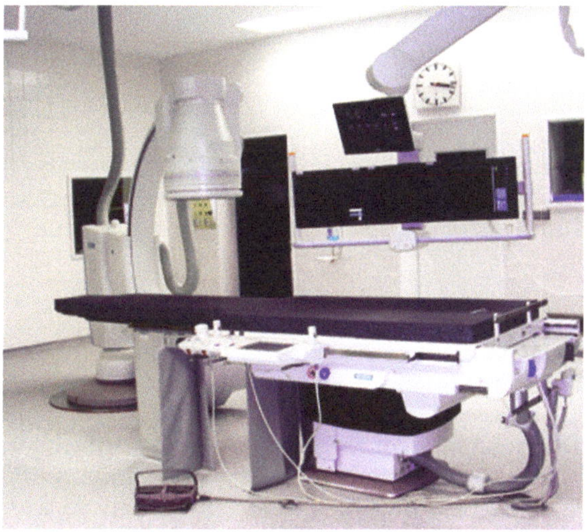

FIG. 5.1 View of the first angiosuite hybrid operating room in Germany, at St. Franziskus Hospital, Münster.

The treatment of patients requiring the chimney endovascular technique requires exposure of at least one upper extremity.[1] Consequently, there is a need to prepare the OR accordingly. Long tables are important because of the introduction of long sheaths, catheters, and introducer systems of the bridging devices. In addition, it is beneficial to have a separate table for the wires required to advance the angiographic catheters and sheaths in the renovisceral aorta and to target side branches.

Fig. 5.3 shows the second hybrid OR at St. Franziskus Hospital. The long tables are prepared for the chimney technique with the upper left extremity, the standard access for single- and double-chimney graft placement.

Fig. 5.4 shows the preparation of the angiosuite OR for the chimney endovascular technique from another

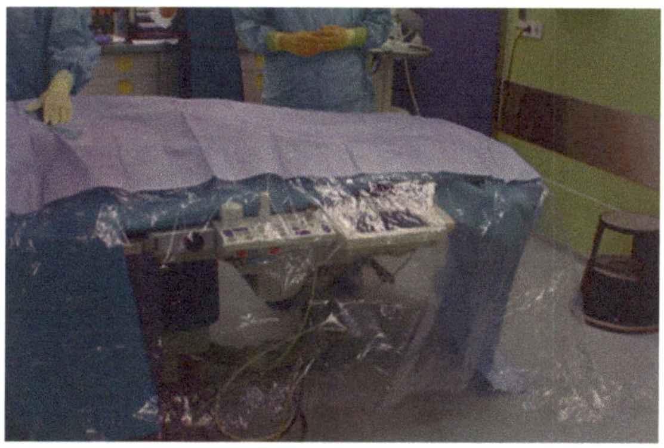

FIG. 5.2 The console at the table improves handling for the operator, especially in challenging pathologies.

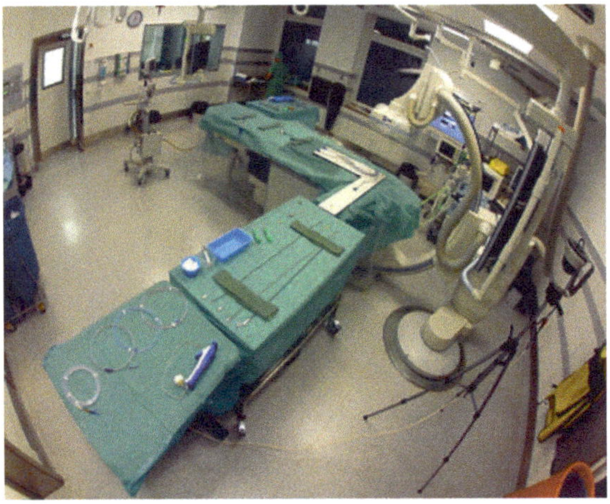

FIG. 5.3 The second angiosuite hybrid OR, Siemens Artis Zee, in Münster, Germany.

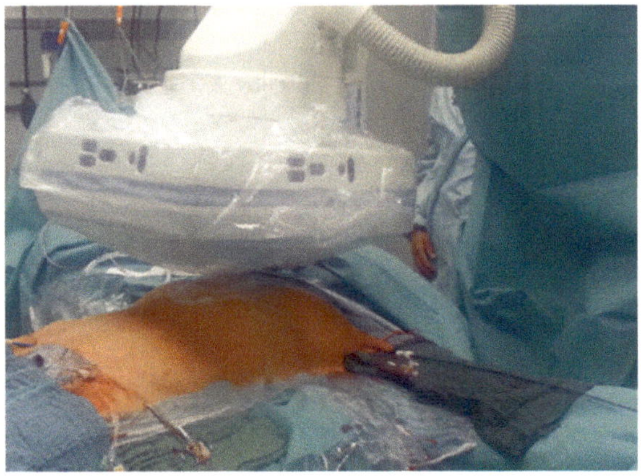

FIG. 5.5 Position of the operator related to the tables and C-arm at the start of the operation.

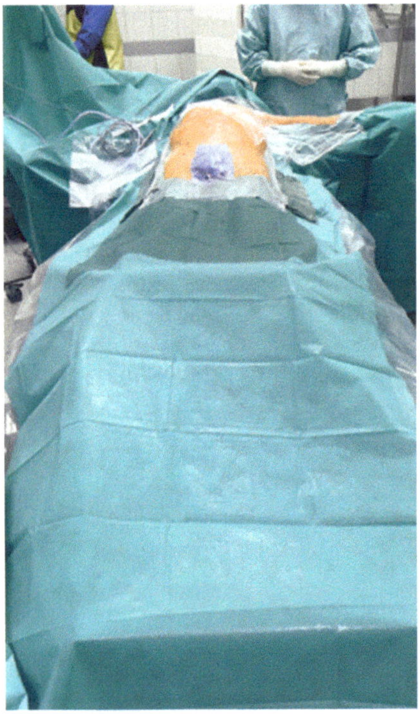

FIG. 5.4 Overview of the hybrid OR for chimney endovascular aortic repair.

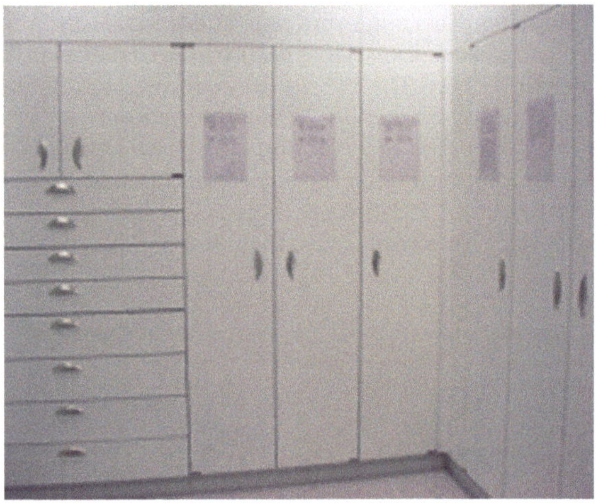

FIG. 5.6 Endovascular materials stock for complex EVAR at St. Franziskus Hospital.

view. The first table has the sheaths and the syringes, and the second table has the wires required for cannulation and advancement of catheters and sheaths. Fig. 5.5 shows the view of the operator, who takes the position on the right side of the patient.

Fig. 5.6 shows the endovascular materials stock at St. Franziskus Hospital, near the hybrid room. Multiple cabinets and lists of contents provide the staff with the logistical means to locate the needed products quickly. Fig. 5.7 depicts the rail systems, which facilitate access to angiographic catheters, balloons, and stents. Fig. 5.8 illustrates baskets and drawer storage for interventional devices.

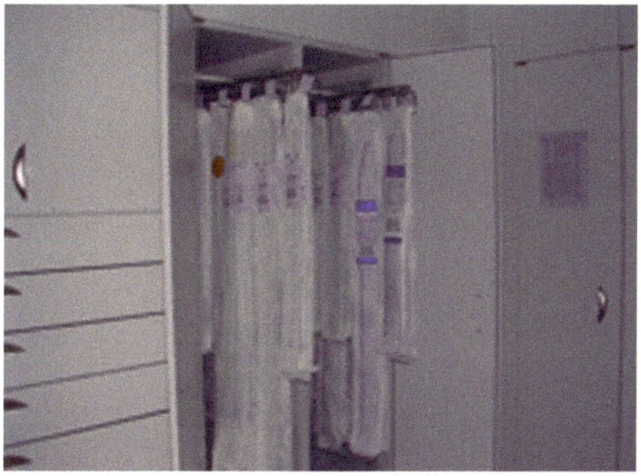

FIG. 5.7 Rail systems improve the overview of endovascular materials.

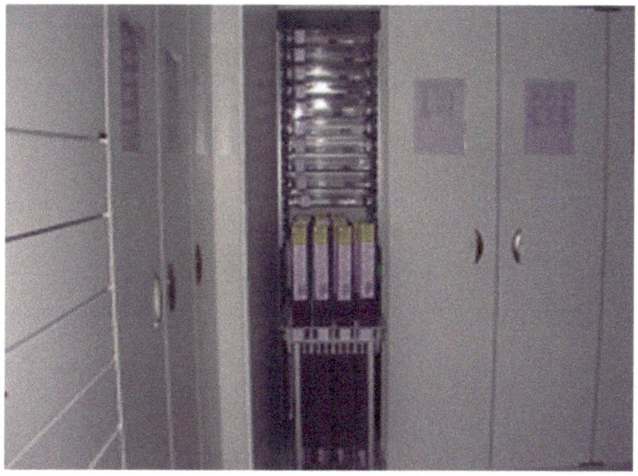

FIG. 5.8 Endovascular storage for complex EVAR.

REFERENCE

1. Torsello G, Donas KP. Endovascular treatment of complex thoracoabdominal and abdominal aortic aneurysms. *Edizioni Minerva Medical*. 2012:1–11.

CHAPTER 6

Overview of Chimney Endovascular Technique

FRANK J. CRIADO • KONSTANTINOS P. DONAS

In an almost 20-year evolution, parallel-graft techniques have emerged as part of the effort to rescue or preserve inadvertently excluded aortic branches during endograft aortic aneurysm repair. Currently, planned vessel-branch revascularization in complex pathologies, including aortic side branches, is more frequently cited as the main reason for their use. Simultaneously, persistent issues related to availability, sizing, procedural complexity, and cost of fenestrated endografts led to wide and expanded use of parallel grafts as a total endovascular solution to complex aortic diseases.

Multiple names have been given to these techniques, including chimneys, snorkels, CHIMPS, periscopes, and sandwich grafts. "Parallel grafts" should be considered as the all-encompassing term that best captures the one feature all branch-preserving conduits share—their intra-aortic parallel course, external to but alongside the main aortic endograft. However, use of the term *chimney graft* was preferred to popularize the technique worldwide.

LITERATURE REVIEW

Roy Greenberg was first to use a chimney stent to revascularize the unintentionally covered right renal artery in 2001 during a complex endovascular aneurysm repair (EVAR) procedure (Table 6.1). The term "snorkel" was suggested before "chimney" by Robert Rutherford, then editor of the *Journal of Vascular Surgery*, during his review of the manuscript by Greenberg et al.[1,2]

In April 2003, Criado[3] placed a bare-metal stent in the left common carotid artery (via retrograde percutaneous puncture in left side of neck) to reestablish antegrade flow after unintentional stent-graft coverage during a thoracic endovascular aortic repair (TEVAR) procedure for treatment of arch aneurysm. The stent was a rescue chimney stent. Larzon et al.[4] performed an almost identical procedure in 2004 to lengthen the proximal fixation zone during TEVAR, but this was done semi-electively and as a component of the procedural plan.

In 2007, Criado[5] documented and illustrated the concept of using longer chimney conduits for arch and abdominal aortic repair. This would become one of the foundations for subsequent developments and new ideas, including the Lachat-Mayer "periscope" technique,[6] first performed by the Zurich group in 2008 to revascularize (from a transfemoral access) the visceral arteries during stent-graft repair of a ruptured thoracoabdominal aortic aneurysm. Lobato's sandwich graft procedures followed, first performed in 2008 for revascularization of the hypogastric artery during abdominal aortic aneurysm (AAA) repair,[7] and in 2009 for the visceral and renal arteries in the context of thoracoabdominal aortic aneurysm treatment.[8]

In 2010, the Münster group published the first significant clinical series (with >10 patients) of treatment for juxtarenal aortic aneurysms facilitated by placement of a single chimney graft in the renal artery.[9] Kasirajan[10] proposed a creative new approach (for treatment of thoracoabdominal aortic aneurysms) using two inverted abdominal bifurcated stent-grafts in the descending thoracic aorta, with subsequent antegrade deployment of additional multiple long conduits extending from the iliac limbs into the visceral arteries. A technical modification of this approach proposed by Silveira et al.[11] obviated the need to use two abdominal grafts.

In 2012, Mestres et al.[12] reported the first in vitro comparison of several chimney-graft EVAR (chEVAR) device combinations. The authors found that gutter formation could be minimized by oversizing the aortic stent-graft by 30% using a combination of Endurant (Medtronic, Santa Rosa, California, USA) and Advanta/i-Cast V12 (Atrium Medical/Maquet, Hudson, New

TABLE 6.1
Historical Milestones for Parallel Grafts (Chimney Technique)

Year	Study	Milestone
2001	Greenberg et al.	First chimney (renal artery)
2003	Criado et al.	First arch-branch chimney (left carotid artery)
2004	Larzon et al.	First planned arch-branch chimney (left carotid artery)
2007	Criado et al.	Suggested/illustrated use of longer chimneys
2008	Malina et al.	Popularization of term *chimneys*
2008	Lachat et al.	Periscope graft (visceral/renal arteries)
2009	Lobato et al.	Sandwich-graft procedure (visceral arteries)
2010	Donas et al.	Report of first clinical series (>10 patients) in treatment of juxtarenal aneurysms
2012	Mestres et al.	In vitro testing of best device combinations for chEVAR
2013	Donas et al.	Clinical results confirming Mestres et al. findings
2015	Donas, Lee, et al.	Worldwide collected experience (PERICLES Registry) results
2016	Donas, Torsello, et al.	PROTAGORAS Study as first attempt to standardize chimney technique
2017	Donas, Criado, et al.	Novel classification (based on causative mechanisms) of type Ia endoleaks and persistent gutters following chEVAR

chEVAR, Chimney-graft endovascular aneurysm repair.

Hampshire, USA) balloon-expandable covered stent, or Excluder with the Viabahn (Gore, Tempe, Arizona, USA) self-expanding covered stent. These findings were reaffirmed in a clinical report of the Münster group with the Zurich colleagues.[13]

In 2013, the same centers also reported the first computed tomography angiography (CTA)–based evaluation of aneurysm sac changes (during 2-year follow-up) in 40 patients.[14] Also in 2013, Lachat et al.[15] reported the first case of transfemoral placement of parallel grafts in the renal arteries, also known as the "lift technique."

CURRENT STATUS

Until recently, parallel-graft techniques lacked a solid evidence foundation, since available clinical data and publications were clearly insufficient to validate their growing use. In recent years, however, several significant studies have provided a much more compelling picture. The greatest impetus came from the international PERICLES Registry in 2015, prompted by the leadership of Frank Veith, Konstantinos Donas, and Jason T. Lee.[16] They laid the foundation for collecting the experience of nine leading chimney-graft centers in Europe and four in the United States. As anticipated, chEVAR (for treatment of complex-anatomy AAA) emerged as the most frequent parallel-graft procedure. The results surpassed expectations, with the relatively low rate of reinterventions for related endoleaks and the patency of the chimney grafts proving very satisfactory overall.

In 2016, the Münster group published the PROTAGORAS Study evaluating the performance of the Endurant abdominal device with balloon-expandable covered chimney stents in 128 patients with complex aortic disease.[17] The results were promising because they underscored the importance of standardization of technique and device choices.

Moreover, in early 2017, the PERICLES Registry collaborators illustrated and proposed a novel classification (based on the causative mechanisms) of type Ia endoleaks and persistent gutters following chEVAR.[18] It is hoped this will further establish the underlying principles to optimize initial results and help develop treatment algorithms for management of complications. Indeed, as widely agreed, these gutters and related endoleaks represent the Achilles' heel of the chEVAR procedure.

The Conformité Européenne (CE) mark granted to chEVAR Endurant with balloon-expandable chimney covered stents in 2016 has elevated their status to approved on-label therapy in specific anatomic conditions.

REFERENCES

1. Greenberg RK, Clair D, Srivastava S, et al. Should patients with challenging anatomy be offered endovascular aneurysm repair? *J Vasc Surg*. 2003;38:990–996.
2. Greenberg RK. *Personal communication (to Criado FJ)*; 2010.
3. Criado FJ. A percutaneous technique for preservation of arch branch patency during thoracic endovascular aortic repair (TEVAR): retrograde catheterization and stenting. *J Endovasc Ther*. 2007;14:54–58.
4. Larzon T, Gruber G, Friberg O, et al. Experiences of intentional carotid stenting in endovascular repair of aortic arch aneurysms—two case reports. *Eur J Vasc Endovasc Surg*. 2005;30:147–151.
5. Criado FJ. Chimney grafts and bare stents: aortic branch preservation revisited. *J Endovasc Ther*. 2007;14: 823–824.
6. Lachat M, Frauenfelder T, Mayer D, et al. Complete endovascular renal and visceral artery revascularization and exclusion of a ruptured type IV thoracoabdominal aortic aneurysm. *J Endovasc Ther*. 2010;17:216–220.
7. Lobato AC. Sandwich technique for aortoiliac aneurysms extending to the internal iliac artery or isolated common/internal iliac artery aneurysms: a new endovascular approach to preserve pelvic circulation. *J Endovasc Ther*. 2011;18:106–111.
8. Lobato AC, Camacho-Lobato L. Endovascular treatment of complex aortic aneurysms using the sandwich technique. *J Endovasc Ther*. 2012;19:691–706.
9. Donas KP, Torsello G, Austermann M, et al. Use of abdominal chimney grafts is feasible and safe: short-term results. *J Endovasc Ther*. 2010;17(5):589–593.
10. Kasirajan K. Branched grafts for thoracoabdominal aneurysms: off-label use of FDA-approved devices. *J Endovasc Ther*. 2011;18:471–476.
11. Silveira PG, Galego GN, Bortoluzzi CT, Franklin RN. RE: "Branched grafts for thoracoabdominal aneurysms: off-label use of FDA-approved devices". *J Endovasc Ther*. 2012;19:130.
12. Mestres G, Uribe JP, Garcia-Madrid C, et al. The best conditions for parallel stenting during EVAR: an in vitro study. *Eur J Vasc Endovasc Surg*. 2012;44(5):468–473.
13. Donas KP, Pecoraro F, Torsello G, et al. Use of covered chimney stents for pararenal aortic pathologies is safe and feasible with excellent patency and low incidence of endoleaks. *J Vasc Surg*. 2012;55(3):659–665.
14. Donas KP, Pecoraro F, Bisdas T, et al. CT angiography at 24 months demonstrates durability of EVAR with the use of chimney grafts for pararenal aortic pathologies. *J Endovasc Ther*. 2013;20(1):1–6.
15. Lachat M, Bisdas T, Rancic Z, et al. Chimney endografting for pararenal aortic pathologies using transfemoral access and the lift technique. *J Endovas Surg*. 2013;20(4):492–497.
16. Donas KP, Lee JT, Lachat M, et al. Collected world experience about the performance of the snorkel/chimney endovascular technique in the treatment of complex aortic pathologies: the PERICLES Registry. *Ann Surg*. 2015;262(3):546–553.
17. Donas KP, Torsello GB, Piccoli G, et al. The PROTAGORAS Study to evaluate the performance of the Endurant stent graft for patients with pararenal pathologic processes treated by the chimney/snorkel endovascular technique. *J Vasc Surg*. 2016;63(1):1–7.
18. Donas KP, Criado FJ, Torsello G, Veith FJ, Minion DJ. PERICLES Registry Collaborators. Classification of chimney EVAR-Related endoleaks: insights from the PERICLES registry. *J Endovasc Ther*. 2017;24(1):72–74.

CHAPTER 7

Sizing of Aortic Endografts in Chimney Technique

STEFANO FAZZINI • KONSTANTINOS P. DONAS • KENNETH OURIEL

In the last decade the endovascular treatment of complex aortic disease was revolutionized with the introduction of the chimney technique, an alternative approach to create an adequate proximal/distal landing zone in the event of an insufficient aneurysm neck. The main issue that determines a successful outcome with the chimney technique is the degree of main endograft oversizing in relation to the parallel grafts. A correct oversizing is crucial to achieve an appropriate balance of the opposing radial forces among the chimney, endograft, and aortic wall. An appropriate amount of oversizing allows the endograft to conform optimally around the stent and avoids both type I endoleaks through large gutters and compression of the parallel graft(s).

Type I endoleaks caused by gutters were often described as the "Achilles' heel" of the chimney procedure. Persistent type I endoleaks requiring reintervention range between 1.6% (PROTAGORAS)[1] and 2.9% (PERICLES).[2] The main reason for this relatively high rate of gutter leaks is a lack of consensus regarding the optimal configuration, combination of devices, and operative technique. It is evident, however, that appropriate planning and selection of devices are crucial to minimize the risk for gutter leaks.

PREOPERATIVE IMAGING

Thoracoabdominal computed tomography angiography (CTA) is essential for preoperative planning. CTA scans should have a thickness of 1 mm to achieve a very high imaging resolution. The imaging should be analyzed using dedicated vascular software for three-dimensional reformatting and centerline reconstructions for exact measurement of vessel length and diameter.

The configuration of the vessels should be carefully studied by multiplanar reconstruction (MPR), particularly at the level of the juxtarenal aorta, to assess the renal and visceral vessels. Also, imaging should include adequate views of the access vessels, such as the iliac and femoral arteries, because these are essential to plan the chimney procedure. Similarly, imaging must include an evaluation of the arch vessels. The subclavian artery is used as the main vessel for the upper extremity access, as well as to rule out high-grade carotid stenoses, which can be a risk for perioperative neurologic complications.

The presence of thrombus in the descending aorta can also be a source of cerebral or visceral embolization. In this context, additional administration of heparin and monitoring of the activated clotting time are strongly recommended.

NEW SEALING LENGTH

The total neck length in the chimney technique is defined as the sum of a seal neck and new neck. The *new neck* is defined as the segment between the proximal fabric edge of the aortic endograft and the orifice of the lowest target vessel in which the chimney graft will be deployed. The *seal neck* reflects the native portion of the infrarenal aortic neck, always shorter than 10 mm and often completely absent. The goal is to have a total neck length of at least 20 mm. This length was required in the PERICLES Registry and the PROTAGORAS Study. Each of the following parameters should be evaluated preoperatively:

1. Identification and characterization of the aortic neck and the involved aortic branches
2. Estimation of the length of the new sealing zone
3. Caliber and length of the infrarenal neck, if present
4. Total aortic length to the bifurcation
5. Anatomic characteristics of the target vessels:
   - Angulation
   - Curvature
   - Origin along the aortic circumference (clock face)
   - Diameter of the branch vessel
   - Length, with consideration of relevant branches that perfuse a significant segment of the kidney or the bowel, and whether these could be overstented after deployment of the chimney graft in the main branch

6. Presence of accessory renal arteries and estimation of the renal mass supplied by the vessel for preoperative decision making, regarding whether overstenting or maintaining perfusion is preferable
7. Descending thoracic aortic and iliac artery tortuosity centerline calculations (mandatory to assess length accurately in tortuous anatomy)
8. Caliber and presence of calcification of the common femoral arteries and the external iliac arteries

PLANNING THE PROCEDURE

Aortic Neck Sizing

Current devices and technical skills have increased the applicability of standard endovascular aneurysm repair (EVAR) to a broad spectrum of patients with aortic aneurysms. Regarding the infrarenal aortic neck, current instructions for use (IFU) include evaluation of not only standard parameters, such as the length and diameter, but also the shape (conical, bubble, or straight) and the angulation (both suprarenal and infrarenal).

Most latest-generation endograft IFUs specify a required neck length of 15 to 20 mm, but lengths of 10 mm may be acceptable when the neck is not severely angulated (<60 degrees). The use of chimney technique to treat patients with an inadequate neck length is based on the creation of a new aortic neck of a similar required length, which is at least a 15-mm sealing zone for an abdominal device.

Aortic Neck Diameter

When choosing the size of the aortic endograft, one must assess the diameter of the pararenal aorta at the intended segment for the deployment of the endoprosthesis. In vitro analysis showed that oversizing of 20% to 30% minimizes the risk for persistent gutter-related endoleaks. This means that the maximum neck diameter in single chimneys should be no more than 30 mm. In this case, an aortic device of 36 mm is at least 30% oversizing. It is important to measure the neck diameter in three parts—proximally, medially, and distally—and use adventitia-to-adventitia (outer wall–to–outer wall) measurements, with exception of the Gore endografts (recommend "inner-to-inner" measurements).

Aortic Neck Angulation and Thrombus

Presence of severe (>60 degrees) infrarenal neck angulation and a conical shape are predictors for early type Ia endoleak. These endoleaks can be reduced if the aortic device can be deployed in a straighter aortic segment, avoiding placement in highly angulated anatomy. The surgeon should adhere to this principle, even if doing so would require additional chimney graft placement into the upper aortic branches.

Calcification and mural thrombus are also factors that predispose to suboptimal deployment of the aortic device, poor wall apposition, and a higher risk of type Ia endoleaks, as in infrarenally deployed endografts.

SIZING OF CHIMNEY GRAFTS

A sealing zone of at least 10-mm length into the aortic side branches is recommended. Usually the diameter of the chimney graft is chosen based on the diameter of the target vessel. For example, a 6-mm chimney graft would be chosen for visceral vessels with a diameter between 5.1–6mm. Placement of a nitinol bare-metal stent in an already-deployed chimney graft lengthens the distal sealing zone while maintaining perfusion of a relevant side branch. The diameter of the additionally deployed nitinol stent is the same as the diameter of the previously deployed chimney graft.

AORTIC BRANCH STENOSIS OR ANGULATION

Severely calcified stenoses of the visceral vessels are associated with a technically demanding procedure. Predilation with a 4-mm balloon catheter can be a good option. Alternatively, the use of the "lift technique"[3] allows the transfemoral placement of self-expanding chimney grafts. This technique permits the creation of a standard chimney configuration from a femoral approach, moving the proximal aspect of the chimney graft cranially after deployment. Fig. 7.1 shows the already-deployed Viabahn self-expanding covered stent in the left renal artery. A short balloon is positioned at the distal aspect of the Viabahn chimney graft to fix its position. The sheath is then advanced cranially to reposition the chimney graft so that its proximal aspect is in a normal chimney configuration, proximal to the branch vessel for antegrade perfusion into the branch.

OVERSIZING OF ABDOMINAL ENDOGRAFT

Four options can be considered to determine the proper amount of oversizing of aortic endografts for the chimney technique: standard oversizing, use of a mathematical formula, in vitro testing, and custom-made oversizing.

Standard Oversizing

The PERICLES Registry and PROTAGORAS Study recommend oversizing between 20% and 30%. This is based on the clinical experience with standard EVAR, with recommendations for 10% oversizing without a chimney graft.

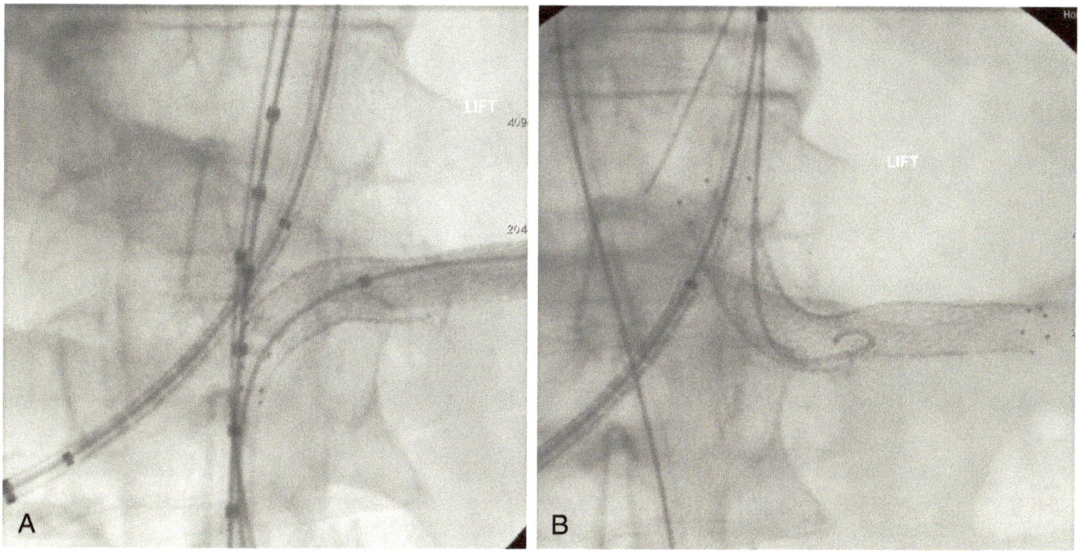

FIG. 7.1 **A, B,** The end result after pushing the proximal portion of the Viabahn chimney graft with the sheath to achieve the final typical chimney configuration.

In order to have enough fabric material to wrap around the chimney grafts, additional oversizing is required.

Mathematical Formula

Lachat suggested during a LINC meeting an elliptic model for the estimation of the appropriate aortic stent-graft diameter. The formula is based on an ellipse configuration with *major diameter* (A) equal to the sum of the mean aortic diameter plus the chimney stent diameters, and *minor diameter* (B) equal to the mean aortic diameter. Mathematically, this is equal to (A + B)/2, if B is the sum of the chimney graft diameters.

Kölbel et al.[4] proposed a mathematical formula using circular segments of the aorta and a single chimney graft of 6–8 mm, concluding that 30% is the best oversizing for a single visceral chimney graft.

In Vitro Testing

According to Mestres et al., 30% is the recommended oversizing when placement of a single chimney graft is planned. The gutters must have the smallest possible area between the chimney and abdominal endografts to minimize the risk for persistent type Ia endoleak. The choice of abdominal endograft also plays an important role.

Two abdominal endografts, the Endurant (Medtronic, Santa Rosa, California, USA) and Excluder (Gore, Tempe, Arizona, USA) were tested with placement of a single chimney graft, either Advanta V12 (Atrium Medical/Maquet, Hudson, New Hampshire, USA) or Viabahn (Gore). The configurations were tested with three different degrees of oversizing: normal (15% oversizing), excessive (30%), and overexcessive (40%). The best results with freedom from chimney graft compression and smallest gutter areas were observed in the combinations of Advanta V12 with a 30% oversized Endurant abdominal device and Viabahn with a 30% oversized Excluder. The increased radial force in the Endurant performs better with a balloon-expandable covered stent, which has also higher radial force compared with self-expanding stents.

Custom-Made Oversizing Technique

"Over-SIRIX" is a new patient-tailored method to select the appropriate abdominal endograft in order to minimize gutter formation and reduce the incidence of type Ia endoleak with the chimney technique (Fig. 7.2). The ideal perimeter is drawn around the chimney graft directly on the CTA (based on Osirix imaging software), where the chimney graft is planned within the axial plane on MPR, at the level of the proximal aspect of the new neck.

To obtain the *ideal* MG sizing ("I-Size"), a formula can be used by adding the *custom* MG sizing ("C-Size") to the *disease* oversizing ("D-Over"). MPR imaging was reassessed on the postoperative CTA to study gutter area and the presence of type Ia endoleak. The formula proposed by the Over-SIRIX method is:

$$\text{C-Size} + \text{D-Over} = \text{I-size}$$

C-Size is measured on CTA (D = C/π; MG sizing = MG perimeter/π), encircling the aortic wall and the

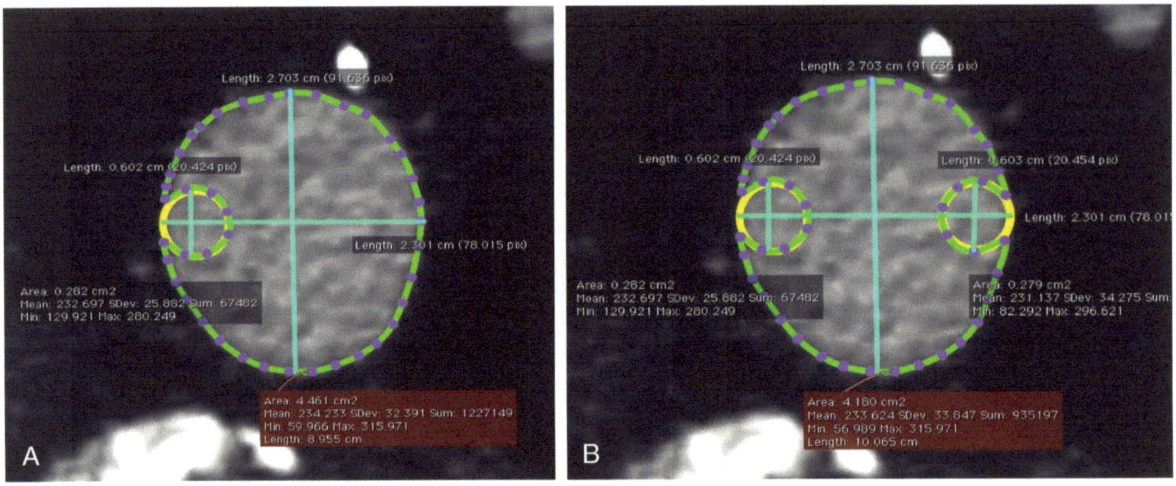

FIG. 7.2 "Over-SIRIX" method. Mean aortic diameter is 25 mm (23 × 27 mm), 6-mm stent. Custom MG sizing is calculated by the length of MG (D = C/π): **A,** 89/π = 28.3; **B,** 100/π = 31.8.

TABLE 7.1
Examples of Aortic Endograft Oversizing with One Chimney Graft

	SIZING				MATERIALS			
	SEALING ZONE		IDEAL MAIN GRAFT		MAIN GRAFT		CHIMNEY GRAFT	
Oversizing Method	**Aortic Neck Diameter**	**Aortic Branch**	**Oversizing**	**Diameter**	**Endurant**	**Excluder**	**Advanta**	**Viabahn**
Standard (20-30%)	25	5	25 + 25%	31.25	32	31	6 x 38/59	6 x 50
Formula (Lachat)	25	5	25 + 3 + 10%	30.8	32	31		6 x 50
Custom ("Over-SIRIX")	25	5	28.3* + 10%		32	31	6 x 38/59	6 x 50

stent area, based on its established diameter (target vessel diameter + 1 mm). Stent shape is drawn as a circle for the smaller stents (5-8 mm; e.g., visceral vessels) or as an oval for larger stents (≥9 mm; e.g., supra-aortic vessels), especially if the stent is self-expanding. D-Over is added for aortic disease (e.g., 10% for aneurysm), and the sum is the I-Size, or ideal MG size.

Tables 7.1 and 7.2 provide examples of aortic endograft oversizing with one or two chimney grafts. Fig. 7.3 to 7.9 illustrate chimney endovascular techniques for oversizing using various combinations of stent-grafts and sizes.

APPROPRIATE COMBINATION OF ABDOMINAL ENDOPROSTHESIS AND CHIMNEY GRAFT

In their in vitro analysis, Mestres et al.[5] concluded that the best combination seems to be either the Endurant and Advanta V12 or the Excluder and Viabahn. The Endurant with Viabahn combination is not recommended because of the risk for covered-stent compression. The Endurant and the Excluder have nitinol-skeleton endografts but have different fixation mechanisms and different radial force at the proximal

TABLE 7.2
Examples of Aortic Endograft Oversizing with Two Chimney Grafts

	SIZING				MATERIALS			
	SEALING ZONE		IDEAL MAIN GRAFT		MAIN GRAFT		CHIMNEY GRAFT	
Oversizing Method	**Aortic Neck Diameter**	**Aortic Branch**	**Oversizing**	**Diameter**	**Endurant**	**Excluder**	**Advanta**	**Viabahn**
Standard (20-30%)	25	5 + 5	25 + 25%	33.75	36	35	6 x 38/59 (double)	6 x 50 (double)
Formula (Lachat)	25	5 + 5	25 + 6 + 10%	34.1	36	35		6 x 50 (double)
Custom ("Over-SIRIX")	25	5 + 5	31.8* + 10%	34.98	36	35	6 x 38/59 (double)	6 x 50 (double)

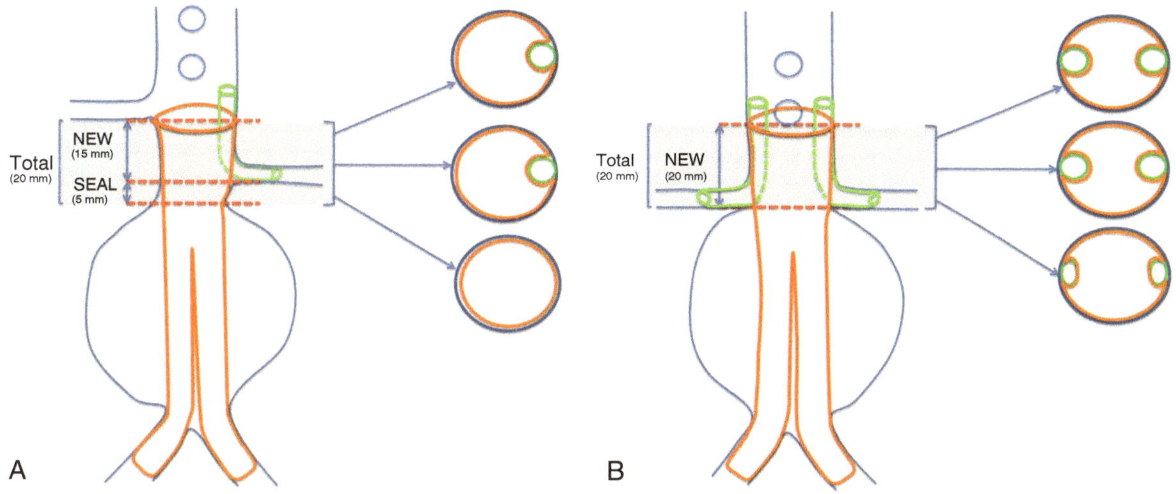

FIG. 7.3 **A,** Single chimney graft (left renal artery). **B,** Double chimney grafts (bilateral renal arteries).

fabric edge, resulting from the presence or absence of suprarenal stents (Table 7.3).

The PROTAGORAS Study first investigated performance of the Endurant stent-graft for patients with pararenal pathologic processes requiring balloon-expandable covered stents in the involved target vessels (chimney grafts). The results were promising, demonstrating a low incidence of type Ia endoleak (1.6%), as well as primary patency of the chimney grafts of 95.7%.

Consequently, at the end of 2016, the Endurant stent-graft (Medtronic) received a Conformité Européenne (CE) mark for the use of chimney grafts in patients with short aortic necks.

LIMITATIONS AND SOLUTIONS

The most important contraindications for the use of chimney-graft EVAR include the following:

- Aortic diameter greater than 29 mm (The largest commercially available endograft diameter is 36 mm.)

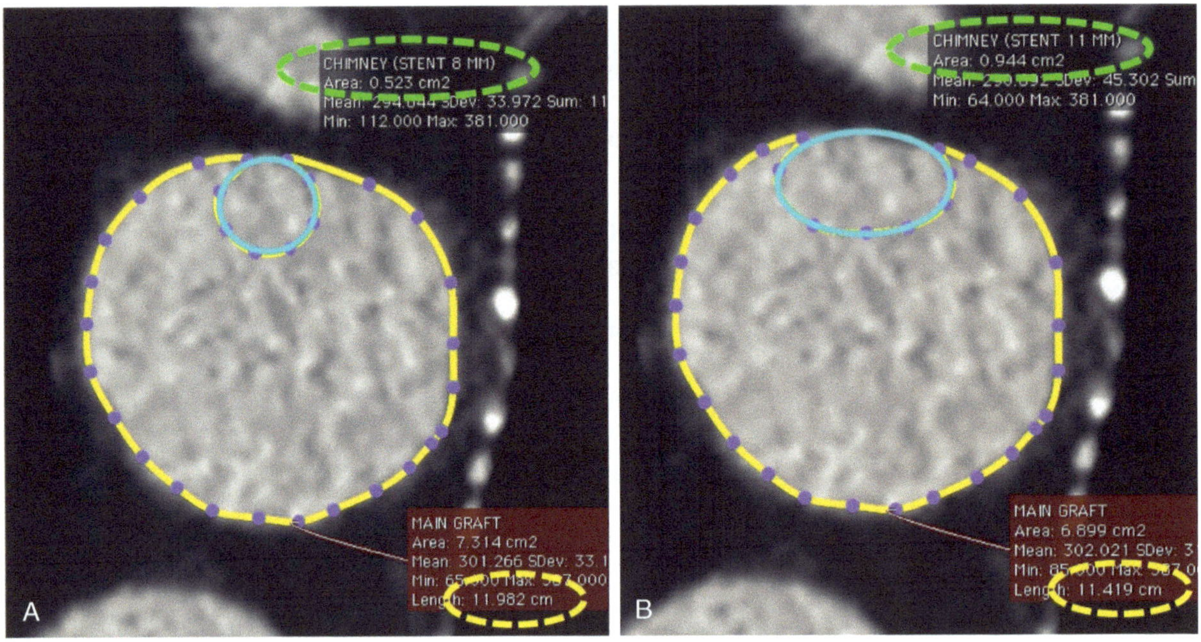

FIG. 7.4 Custom MG sizing. **A,** Larger MG for shorter stent, and **B,** shorter MG for larger stent, depending on stent shape (oval for stent ≥9 mm).

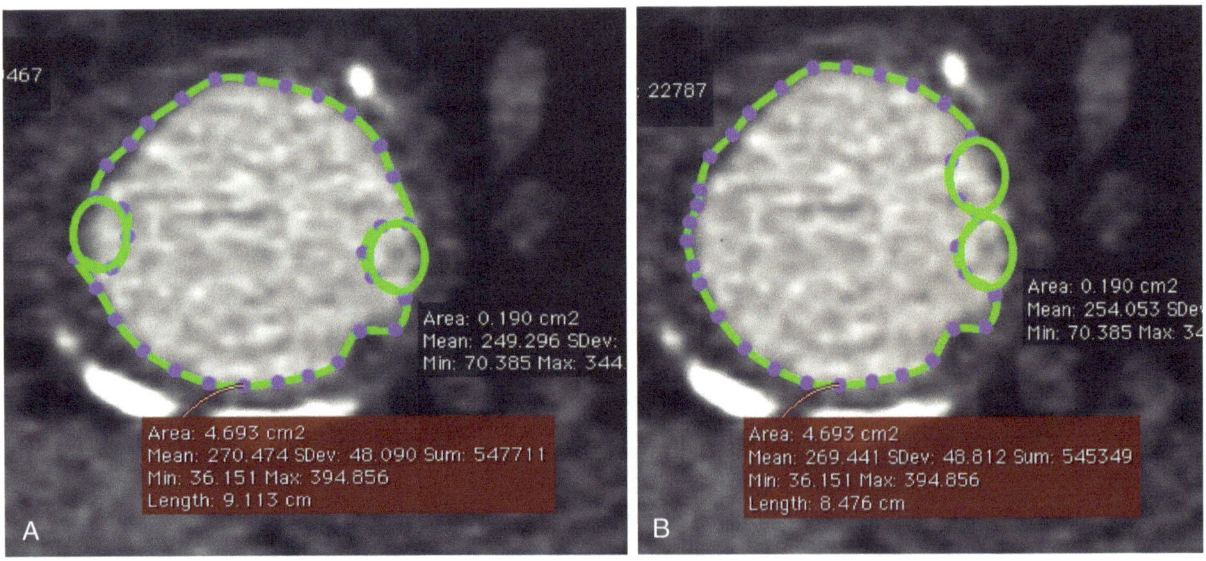

FIG. 7.5 Two chimney grafts at 5 mm (stent area = $r^2 \times \pi = 2.5^2 \times \pi = 19.6\ mm^2$). **A,** Opposite side of the aorta; custom MG sizing is larger (D = C/π = 91/π = 29 mm). **B,** Same side of the aorta; custom MG sizing is lower (D = C/π = 85/π = 27 mm).

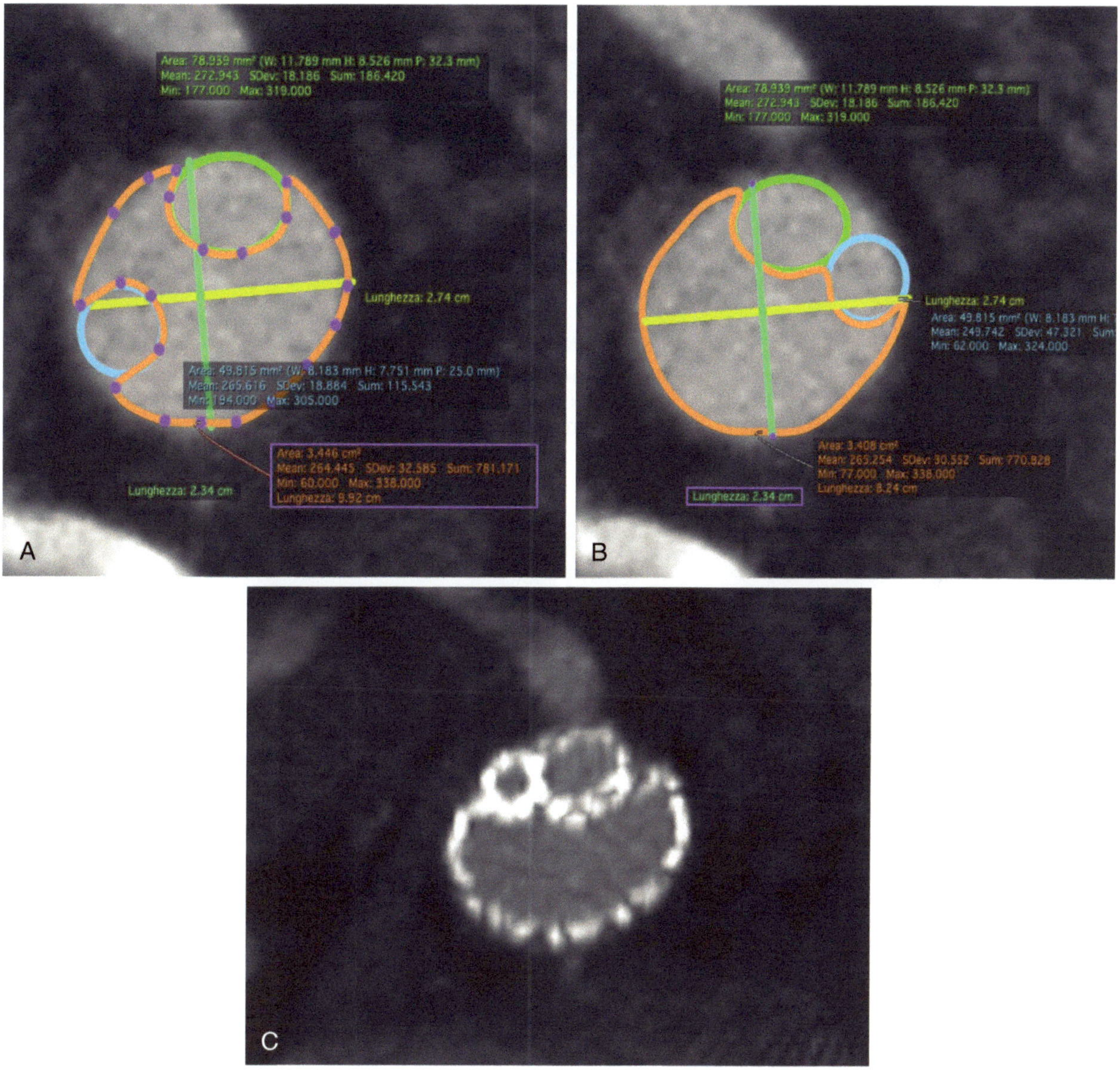

FIG. 7.6 Two chimney grafts at 10 mm (stent area= $5^2 \times \pi = 78$ mm²) and 8 mm (stent area = $4^2 \times \pi = 50$ mm²). **A,** Opposite side of the aorta; custom MG sizing is larger (D = C/π = 99/π = 31 mm). **B,** Same side of the aorta; custom MG sizing is lower (D = C/π = 82/π = 26 mm). **C,**

- Aortic branch diameter less than 4 mm (The smallest covered-stent diameter is 5 mm.)

In addition, the following conditions are associated with a high risk for complications:

1. Extensive mural thrombus in the descending thoracic aorta and left subclavian artery, associated with high risk for neurologic complications
2. Upward orientation of the renal arteries
3. Severe stenosis of the renal arteries
4. Narrow pararenal aortic segment, with a diameter of 23 mm or less
5. Orifice of the renal arteries and superior mesenteric artery at the same level

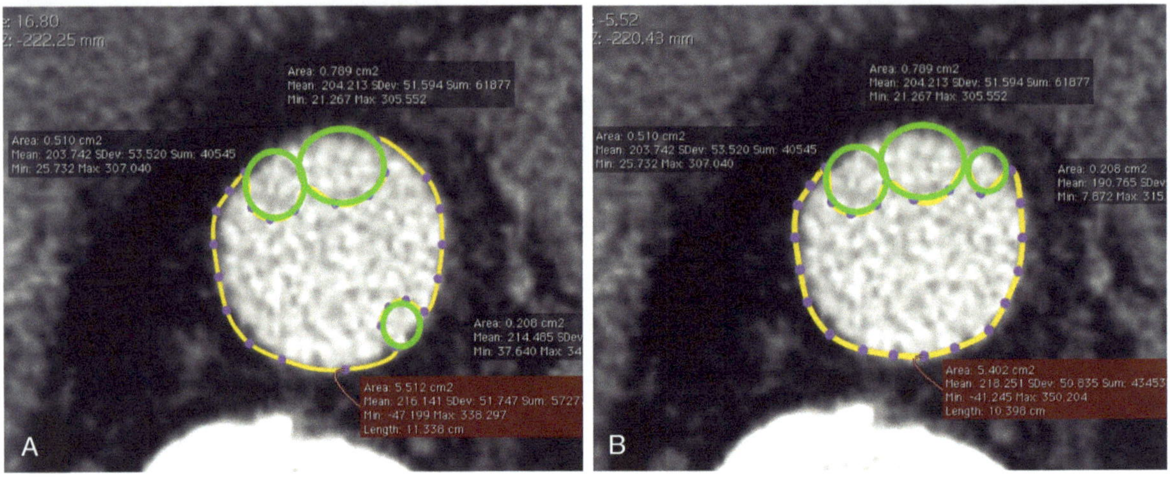

FIG. 7.7 Three chimney grafts at 5 mm (stent area = $r^2 \times \pi = 2.5^2 \times \pi = 19.6$ mm^2), 8 mm (stent area = $r^2 \times \pi = 4^2 \times \pi = 50$ mm^2), and 10 mm (stent area = $r^2 \times \pi = 5^2 \times \pi = 78$ mm^2). **A,** Opposite side of the aorta; custom MG sizing is larger ($D = C/\pi = 113/\pi = 36$ mm). **B,** Same side of the aorta; custom MG sizing is lower ($D = C/\pi = 103/\pi = 33$ mm).

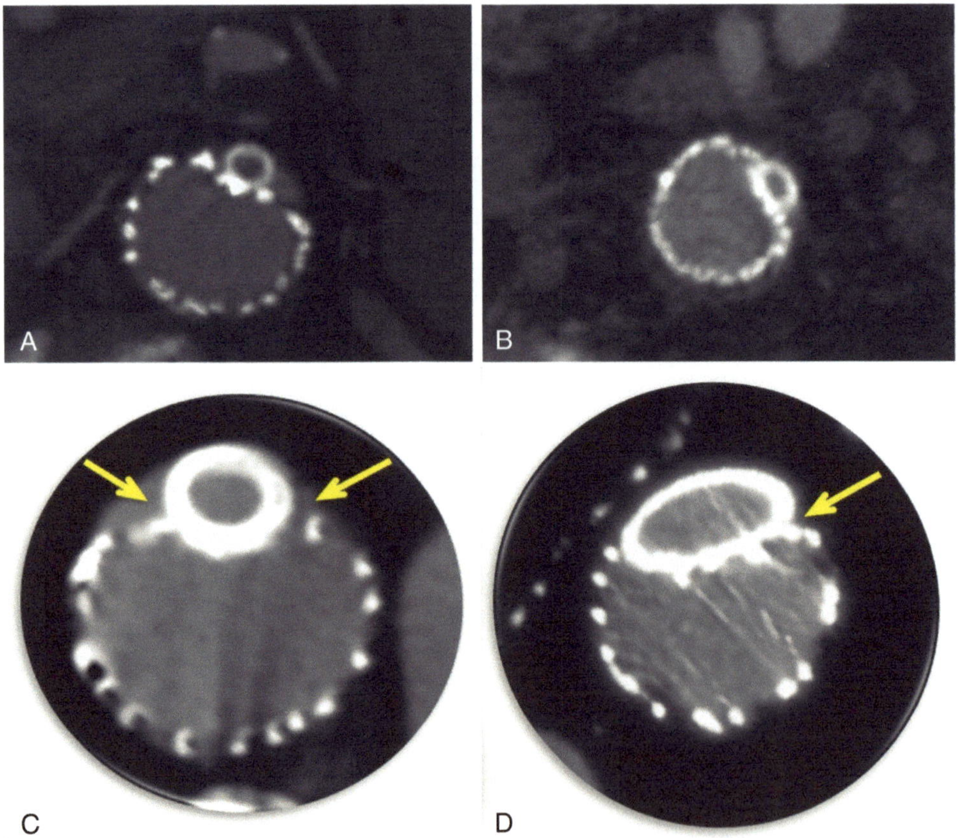

FIG. 7.8 **A,** MG with downsizing (wide gutters). **B,** MG with right sizing (no gutters). **C,** Wide gutters with small stent (circle shape). **D,** Small gutters with large stent (oval shape).

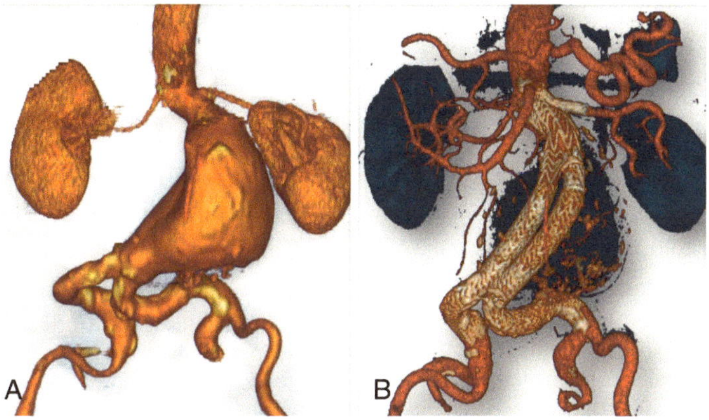

FIG. 7.9 **A, B,** Example of Gore + Viabahn.

TABLE 7.3
Appropriateness of Abdominal Endografts and Chimney Grafts

	MAIN ABDOMINAL GRAFT		CHIMNEY GRAFT	
Features	**Endurant (Medtronic)**	**Excluder (Gore)**	**Advanta V12 (Atrium)**	**Viabahn (Gore)**
Endoskeleton	Nitinol	Nitinol	Stainless steel	Nitinol
Covered materials	Polyester	ePTFE	ePTFE	ePTFE
Fixation	Suprarenal (M-shaped stent)	Infrarenal (barbs)	—	—
Deployment	Precise positioning adjustments	Repositionable	Balloon expandable	Self-expanding
Visibility	+++	+++	+++	+
Trackability	+++	++	+++	+++
Technology	Hydrophilic coating	C3 delivery system	PTFE film–covering technology	Heparin bioactive surface
Sizing (diameter/length, mm)	23-36	25/35	22/32/38/59	50-100-150
French size	18-20F (OD)	16-18F (ID)	7F	8F

ePTFE, Expandable polytetrafluoroethylene; *OD,* outer diameter; *ID,* inner diameter.

DISCUSSION AND CONCLUSIONS

The main goal of the chimney technique is to extend the sealing zone in patients with pathologic processes resulting in a short infrarenal neck for standard EVAR. Extension of the sealing zone allows aneurysm exclusion and preservation of blood flow to the aortic side branches in patients who would otherwise require fenestrated repair or open surgery.

Conceptually, the chimney technique wraps the abdominal device around the chimney grafts to create a parallel and harmonic configuration. Ideally, this will lead to smooth apposition to the aortic wall, without chimney graft compression or gutter formation. The Achilles' heel of the technique, however, remains gutter-related endoleaks. Importantly, more than half of these leaks resolve spontaneously in follow-up, probably from the "low-flow" endoleaks in the majority of these cases.

The presence of a native sealing neck, even if very short, is fundamental to achieve sealing, representing a cul-de-sac for a potentially dangerous gutter. In the absence of this, the sealing of flow in the gutter is proportional to the length and inversely proportional to the gutter area. Thus an ideal aortic neck for chimney grafts is one that has good endoluminal morphology (not calcified) and is relatively long, possibly including only one or two aortic branch vessels. The number of grafts also may influence the success of the technique; the greater the number of chimney grafts, the higher the risk for gutter endoleaks, graft compression, and other complications. Endoleaks and chimney grafts are related, and a classification has been proposed to evaluate different outcomes, such as excessive or insufficient oversizing and inadequate sealing zone.

In conclusion, achieving successful results for the chimney technique depends on a careful evaluation of all chimney graft parameters, with precise, custom planning and the right choice of devices.

REFERENCES

1. Donas KP, Torsello GB, Piccoli G, et al. The PROTAGORAS Study to evaluate the performance of the Endurant stent graft for patients with pararenal pathologic processes treated by the chimney/snorkel endovascular technique. *J Vasc Surg*. 2016;63(1):1–7.
2. Donas KP, Lee JT, Lachat M, et al. Collected world experience about the performance of the snorkel/chimney endovascular technique in the treatment of complex aortic pathologies: the PERICLES Registry. *Ann Surg*. 2015;262(3):546–553.
3. Lachat M, Bisdas T, Rancic Z, et al. Chimney endografting for pararenal aortic pathologies using transfemoral access and the lift technique. *J Endovasc Ther*. 2013;20(4):492–497.
4. Kölbel T, Carpenter SW, Taraz A, et al. How to calculate the main aortic graft-diameter for a chimney-graft. *J Cardiovasc Surg (Torino)*. 2016;57(1):66–71.
5. Mestres G, Uribe JP, García-Madrid C, et al. The best conditions for parallel stenting during EVAR: an in vitro study. *Eur J Vasc Endovasc Surg*. 2012;44(5):468–473.

CHAPTER 8

Procedural Steps in Chimney Technique

KONSTANTINOS P. DONAS

The chimney technique in endovascular aneurysm repair (EVAR) is performed in a hybrid operating room under fluoroscopic control (e.g., Axiom Artis FA and Artis Zee; Siemens Medical Solutions, Forchheim, Germany; at St. Franziskus Hospital, Münster) and under general anesthesia. A totally percutaneous bilateral femoral approach is used, with Prostar XL 10F vascular closure devices (Abbott Vascular, Abbott Park, Illinois, USA).

The left brachial artery for a single chimney graft, or the axillary artery for double chimneys, is surgically exposed for access from the upper extremity (Fig. 8.1). When more than two chimney grafts are planned, the right axillary artery is also exposed.

The next step is the puncture of the axillary artery. As shown in Fig. 8.2, double puncture of the axillary artery, with 1 to 2 cm between the two puncture sites, is used for placement of 2 chimney grafts. The benefit for using this technique is the avoidance of bilateral cannulation and catheterization of the entire aortic arch, minimizing the risk for cerebrovascular events.

The next step is the advance of a 7-French (7F) sheath. With this size of sheath, it is possible to insert balloon-expandable covered stents in the renovisceral vessels with a diameter between 5 and 7 mm. In our institution in Münster, we routinely use the 7F shuttle sheath (Cook, Bloomington, Indiana, USA) (Fig. 8.3).

Chimney grafts are advanced into the renovisceral aortic segment after target vessel cannulation with a 5F catheter. A Rosen wire (Infiniti Medical, Malibu, California, USA), which has an atraumatic tip to prevent iatrogenic injury to the kidney parenchyma, is advanced, followed by placement of a 7F sheath vessel, with secure positioning in the target artery. Deployment of the main aortic stent-graft precedes chimney implantation.

The Endurant abdominal stent-graft (Medtronic, Santa Rosa, California, USA) is routinely used at our institution. We also routinely use balloon-expandable covered stents (BECS, Advanta/iCASTV12; Atrium Medical/Maquet, Hudson, New Hampshire, USA) for the chimney grafts.

Additional alignment of the chimneys with placement of a bare-metal stent (SMART, Cordis, Fremont, California, USA, or Complete, Medtronic) can be performed to improve the flexibility and transition of the chimney stent in angulated target vessels. After the deployment of the chimney grafts, balloon molding should be always performed to ensure adequate seal at the newly created proximal neck and to minimize the "gutters."

Fig. 8.4 illustrates an abdominal aortic aneurysm with a short, angulated neck and angulated left renal artery treated with chimney-graft placement into the left renal artery and EVAR.

Fig. 8.5 presents the concept of lining of chimney grafts with self-expanding bare-metal stents. The bare stent creates a funnel at the distal edge of the rigid, balloon-expandable covered stent. This inhibits the formation of neointimal hyperplasia and stenosis of the chimney graft at the distal edge and also provides a more parallel configuration between the chimney and the abdominal endograft, a configuration associated with better patency rates.

The limitation of this technique is related to the use of additional devices within a chimney device 6 mm in diameter, a scenario that can cause occlusion because of a reduction in lumen size. No robust evidence exists in the literature regarding this issue.

LITERATURE REVIEW

The PERICLES Registry is currently the largest series on the real-world use of chimney-graft EVAR (chEVAR), including 517 patients with pararenal aortic pathologies. Significant aneurysm sac regression, chimney graft primary patency rate of 94.1%, and low incidence of persistent or new, late type Ia endoleaks requiring reintervention confirm reproducible results and the broad applicability of this approach for most surgeons.

Since the first publications on the deployment of covered stents into aortic side branches parallel to and outside the main abdominal endografts, issues such as

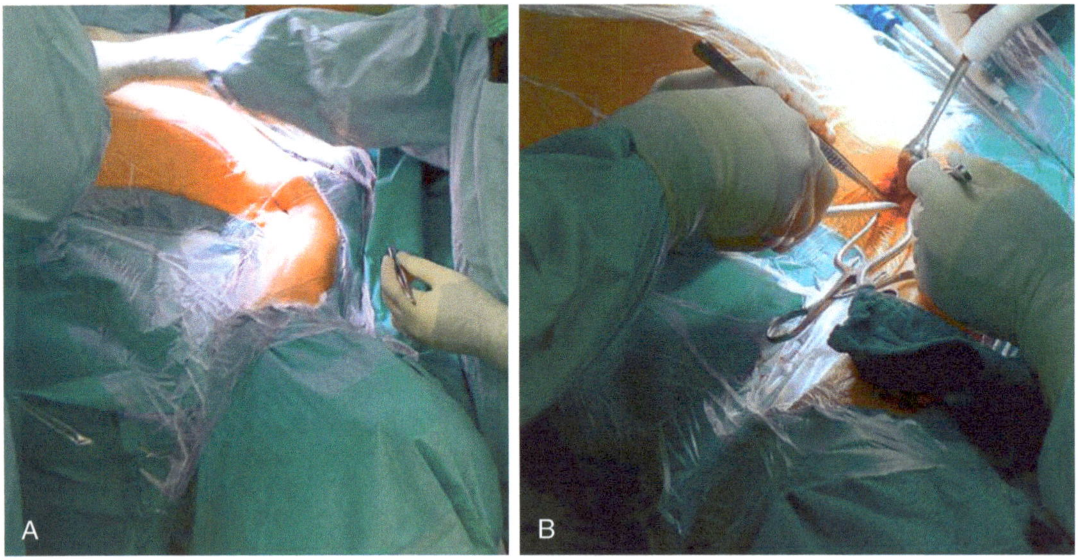

FIG. 8.1 **A, B,** Localization of the incision for axillary artery exposure.

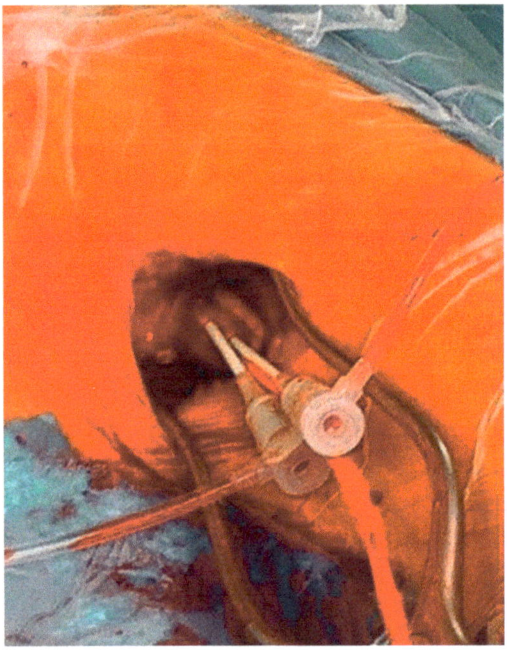

FIG. 8.2 Double-puncture technique of the axillary artery introducing two short, 5F sheaths. This is the preferred approach in our Münster, Germany, institution for cases in need of double–chimney graft placement.

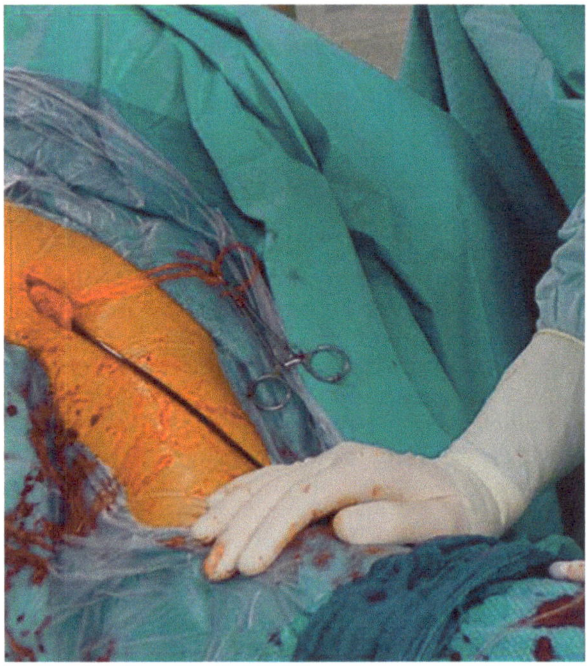

FIG. 8.3 The advance of a 7F shuttle sheath.

the clinical importance of gutter-associated endoleaks remain.[1-18] The PERICLES Registry demonstrated that the need for secondary procedures is rare in the presence of a sufficient proximal landing-zone length of more than 20 mm. The majority of intraoperative type Ia endoleaks disappeared after prolonged kissing-balloon angioplasty between the abdominal and chimney

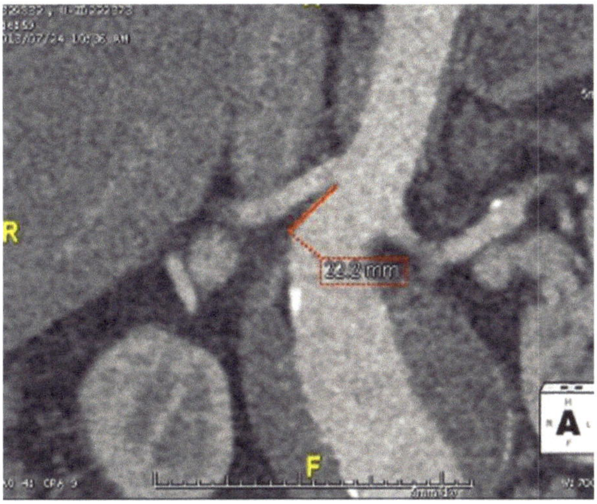

FIG. 8.4 An abdominal aortic aneurysm with a short angulated neck and angulated left renal artery treated with chimney-graft placement into the left renal artery and EVAR.

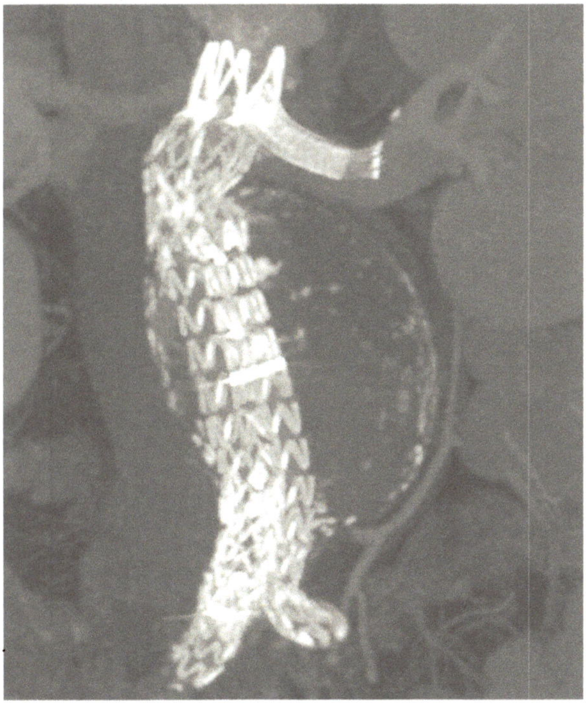

FIG. 8.5 Lining chimney grafts with self-expanding bare-metal stents.

stent-grafts or after additional cuff placement. When persistent type Ia endoleaks are present on postoperative computed tomography (CT), meticulous follow-up is mandatory to evaluate the aneurysm sac diameter.

The PERICLES Registry demonstrates broad feasibility of the chimney technique with the most common available abdominal endografts, culminating in significant shrinkage of the aneurysm sac. However, more data and multivariate analyses are necessary to identify the recommended combinations of abdominal devices and chimney grafts that can minimize the risk of gutters and achieve durable results.[17–18]

The PROTAGORAS Study showed that standard use of the Endurant device with balloon-expandable covered stents as chimneys is associated with significant aneurysm sac regression and low incidence of new type Ia endoleaks that required reintervention. In addition, midterm patency of the chimney grafts appears promising and comparable to the patency of bridging devices after f-EVAR.

REFERENCES

1. Greenberg RK, Clair D, Srivastava S, et al. Should patients with challenging anatomy be offered endovascular aneurysm repair? *J Vasc Surg*. 2003;38(5):990–996.
2. Criado FJ. Chimney grafts and bare stents: aortic branch preservation revisited. *J Endovasc Ther*. 2007;14:823–824.
3. Coscas R, Kobeiter H, Desgranges P, et al. Technical aspects, current indications, and results of chimney graft for juxtarenal aortic aneurysms. *J Vasc Surg*. 2011;53:1520–1526.
4. Allaqaband S, Jan MF, Bajwa T. "The chimney graft": a simple technique for endovascular repair of complex juxtarenal abdominal aortic aneurysms in no-option patients. *Catheter Cardiovasc Interv*. 2010;75:1111–1115.
5. Donas KP, Pecoraro F, Torsello G, et al. CT angiography at 24 months demonstrates durability of EVAR with the use of chimney grafts for pararenal aortic pathologies. *J Endovasc Ther*. 2013;20:1–6.
6. Lachat M, Veith FJ, Pecoraro F, et al. Chimney and periscope grafts observed over 2 years after their use to revascularize 169 renovisceral branches in 77 patients with complex aortic aneurysms. *J Endovasc Ther*. 2013;20:597–605.
7. Lee JT, Greenberg JI, Dalman RL. Early experience with the snorkel technique for juxtarenal aneurysms. *J Vasc Surg*. 2012;55:935–946.
8. Donas KP, Pecoraro F, Torsello G, et al. Use of covered chimney stents for pararenal aortic pathologies is safe and feasible with excellent patency and low incidence of endoleaks. *J Vasc Surg*. 2012;55:659–665.
9. Donas KP, Torsello G, Bisdas T, et al. Early outcomes for fenestrated and chimney endografts in the treatment of pararenal aortic pathologies are not significantly different: a systematic review with pooled data analysis. *J Endovasc Ther*. 2012;19(6):723–728.
10. Pecoraro F, Pfammatter T, Mayer D, et al. Multiple periscope and chimney grafts to treat ruptured thoracoabdominal and pararenal aortic aneurysms. *J Endovasc Ther*. 2011;18:642–649.

11. Chaikof EL, Blankensteijn JD, Harris PL, et al. Reporting standards for endovascular aortic aneurysm repair. *J Vasc Surg*. 2002;35:1048–1060.
12. Schiro A, Antoniou GA, Ormesher D, et al. The chimney technique in endovascular aortic repair: late ruptures after successful single renal chimney stent grafts. *Ann Vasc Surg*. 2013:1–9.
13. Katsargyris A, Oikonomou K, Klonaris C. Comparison of outcomes with open, fenestrated, and chimney graft repair of juxtarenal aneurysms: are we ready for a paradigm shift? *J Endovasc Ther*. 2013;20(2):159–169.
14. Knowles M, Nation DA, Timaran DE, et al. Upper extremity access for fenestrated endovascular aortic aneurysm repair is not associated with increased morbidity. *J Vasc Surg*. 2015;61(1):80–87.
15. Lachat M, Bisdas T, Rancic Z, et al. Chimney endografting for pararenal aortic pathologies using transfemoral access and the lift technique. *J Endovasc Ther*. 2013;20(4): 492–497.
16. Treitl KM, König C, Reiser M, et al. Complications of transbrachial arterial access for peripheral endovascular interventions. *J Endovasc Ther*. 2015;22:63–70.
17. Scali S, Feezor RJ, Chang CK, et al. Critical analysis of results after chimney endovascular aortic aneurysm repair raises cause for concern. *J Vasc Surg*. 2014;2:1–10.
18. Mestres G, Uribe JP, Garcia-Madrid C, et al. The best conditions for parallel stenting during EVAR: an in vitro study. *Eur J Vasc Endovasc Surg*. 2012;44:468–473.

CHAPTER 9

Sizing of Fenestrated Endografts

KONSTANTINOS P. DONAS • MARTIN AUSTERMANN

Preoperative drawing of the aneurysm's anatomic characteristics, with a focus on access and the neck, is our standard approach in endovascular aneurysm repair (EVAR), based on the Osirix planning program. Presents a sketch based on analysis of the patient's vascular anatomy and characteristics, which is always done by the operator.

For the planning of fenestrated endografts, a 1-mm-thick, multislice computed tomography (CT) scan and modern software with the option of centerline reconstruction are necessary.[1] Creation and correction of the centerline with the "racing line" enables the operator to visualize how the endograft will align in the aorta after the deployment (Fig. 9.1). Using the stretched reconstruction, the distances between the visceral arteries and renal arteries can be exactly measured, and the clock position of the target vessels can be determined accurately.

The next step is the selection of a fenestrated or branched endograft. In juxtarenal aneurysms with an inner aortic diameter of 30 mm at the level of the visceral and renal arteries, a fenestrated stent-graft is preferred.[2] The goal is to achieve contact of the device with the aortic wall at the level of the fenestrations, to reduce the risk of endoleaks.[2]

Challenging anatomies with kinking of the aorta at the level of the fenestrations are outside the instructions for use and make the planning demanding. Imaging demonstrates whether the anatomy is suitable for fenestrated endovascular repair (Fig. 9.2).

One option is to taper the graft down at the region of the fenestrations, creating more space between the fenestrations and the ostia of the vessels. This simplifies cannulation of the target vessels.

Use of covered stents as a bridging device is the first choice, especially if there is no aortic wall apposition of the graft at this level. The goal is always to deploy the first two thirds of the bridging device in the target vessel and the distal portion in the fenestrated endograft. Also, flaring of the device is performed with an oversized balloon. This technique stabilizes the position of the device in the fenestrated endograft and target vessel.

Standard design for the treatment of juxtarenal aneurysms is an endograft with three fenestrations and one scallop. The diameter of the superior mesenteric artery (SMA) fenestration is 8 mm in most patients, and the diameter of the renal artery fenestrations is usually 6 × 6 mm or 6 × 8 mm. All fenestrations should be secured by placement of covered stents. A preloaded catheter in one of the vessels (frequently the SMA) facilitates

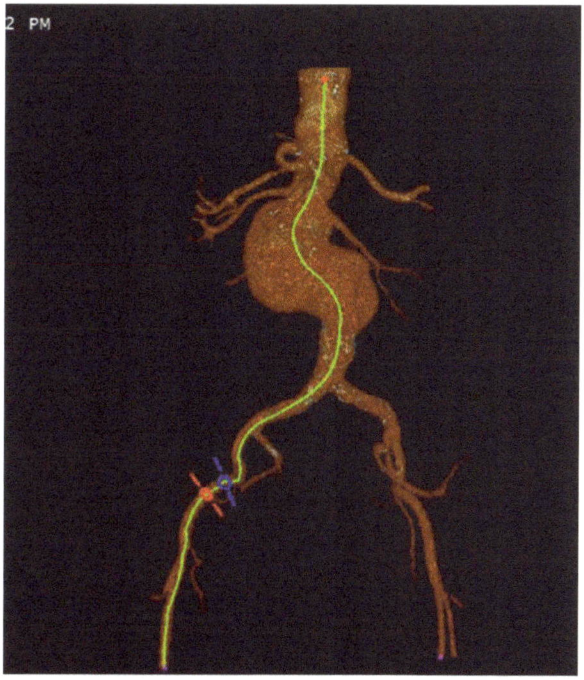

FIG. 9.1 The "racing line" shows how the endograft will align in the aorta after device deployment.

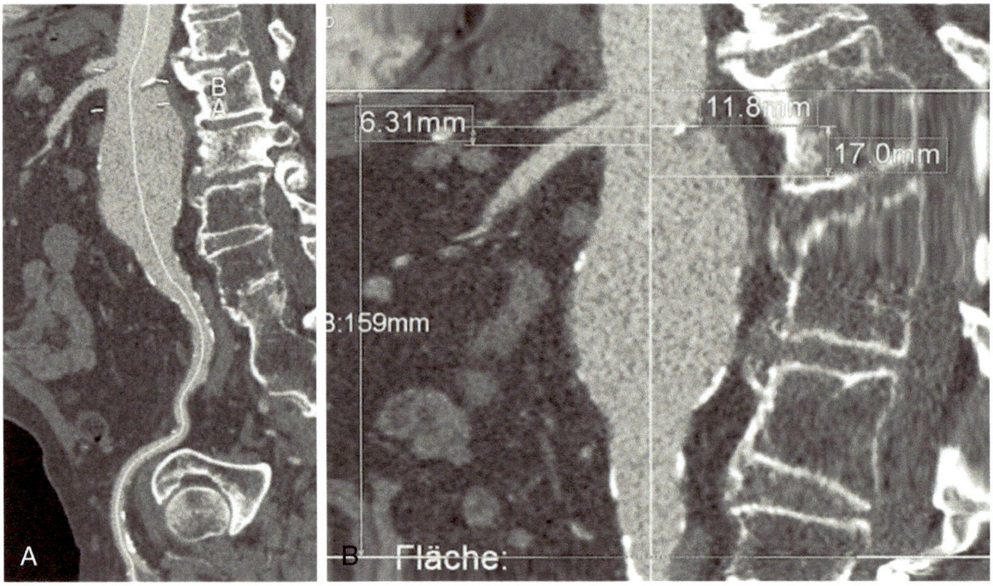

FIG. 9.2 **A, B,** Images demonstrate a suitable anatomy for fenestrated endovascular repair.

access to the fenestrations and represents the standard technique in our Münster, Germany, institution.

In most cases the fenestrated portion of the endograft is a tube and should be oversized by 15% to 25% at the level of the sealing zone. The distal end of the graft should be 22 mm in diameter, so that an off-the-shelf bifurcated graft can be used as the distal component.

REFERENCES

1. Macía I, de Blas M, Legarreta JH, et al. Standard and fenestrated endograft sizing in EVAR planning: description and validation of a semi-automated 3D software. *Comput Med Imaging Graph*. 2016;50:9–23.
2. Austermann M, Torsello G. Planning fenestrated and branched endografts. In: Torsello G, Donas KP, eds. *Endovascular Treatment of Complex Aortic and Thoracoabdominal Aneurysms*. Edizioni Minerva Medical; 2012:19–31.

CHAPTER 10

Fenestrated Endografting for Pararenal Aneurysms

KONSTANTINOS P. DONAS • THEODOSIOS BISDAS • MARTIN AUSTERMANN

The Zenith (Cook Medical, Brisbane, Australia) fenestrated stent-graft (FSG) was developed based on individual patient aneurysm and renal vessel morphology. It is a Conformité Européenne (CE) mark–approved product, with the corresponding preclinical and clinical testing. Despite widespread commercial availability, the use and application of FSGs require advanced technical skills, radiologic imaging and the largest published experience.[1,2]

Particularly demanding parts of the procedure are the catheterization of the target vessels through the fenestrations and subsequent advancement of the 6-French (6F) to 8F sheaths into each vessel. In addition, in patients with calcified and tortuous access vessels, the use of a 22F sheath for the main body and large-bore sheaths through the contralateral iliac artery may be hazardous. Sheath-related complications culminating in lower-limb ischemia are more common in patients with small or diseased iliac and femoral arteries.

To overcome such technical difficulties, a new, modified fenestrated endograft was developed. The new system includes a preloaded wire for easier catheterization of both renal arteries through a lower-profile delivery system (20F instead of 22F).[1]

CASE PRESENTATION

A 74-year-old male patient presented with a juxtarenal aortic aneurysm 65 mm in diameter (Fig. 10.1). The patient had severe comorbidities, including cardiac disease with previous coronary artery bypass, severe chronic obstructive pulmonary disease (COPD), and a history of nicotine abuse and arterial hypertension.

Fig. 10.2 illustrates the preloaded, single, extra-length nitinol wire and its path from the control handle through the center of the stent-graft. The wire passes through the "pusher" directly into the lumen of the graft at its distal end. It then exits from the renal fenestration, passes through the fabric to the other side and then through the contralateral renal fenestration, returning into the delivery system. In addition, the company provides a specific 4.1F braided beacon-tip catheter (Curly-Q, Cook Medical) that facilitates easy catheterization of both renal arteries by keeping the preloaded wire in place, thus stabilizing the introducer sheath.

The procedure was performed in a hybrid operating room under fluoroscopic control (Axiom Artis FA; Siemens Medical Solutions, Forchheim, Germany). Under general anesthesia a percutaneous approach was used with the Prostar XL 10F vascular closure device (Abbott Vascular, Redwood City, California, USA). In case of small or stenotic iliac vessels, a 10-mm bypass from the common iliac to the superficial femoral artery can facilitate stent-graft insertion and implantation.

A 20F sheath was passed into the femoral artery for introduction of the main body. Before delivery of the main stent-graft, a 14F sheath was advanced into the contralateral external iliac artery, and three 5F sheaths were introduced through its valve (Fig. 10.3). Through each 5F sheath, a separate Shepherd Hook catheter (Mayo Healthcare, Rosebery, Australia) was parked into each target vessel: superior mesenteric artery (SMA) and both renal arteries. Fig. 10.4 shows the precannulation of the left renal artery. In our experience, this maneuver facilitates orientation and correct positioning of the main graft without repeated angiography for target-vessel catheterization.

The catheters were removed from each target vessel after each was successfully catheterized with a Rosen wire through the respective fenestrations. Proper orientation of the proximal graft component was controlled by fluoroscopy using gold markers (anterior, posterior, and tick marker). The graft was then advanced into the aorta over a Lunderquist wire (Cook Medical) under fluoroscopic visualization until the fenestrations were just above the ostium of the precatheterized target vessels. The outer sheath was withdrawn until the stent-graft assumed a diamond-like shape. After adjustment of the rotation, the sheath was completely withdrawn.

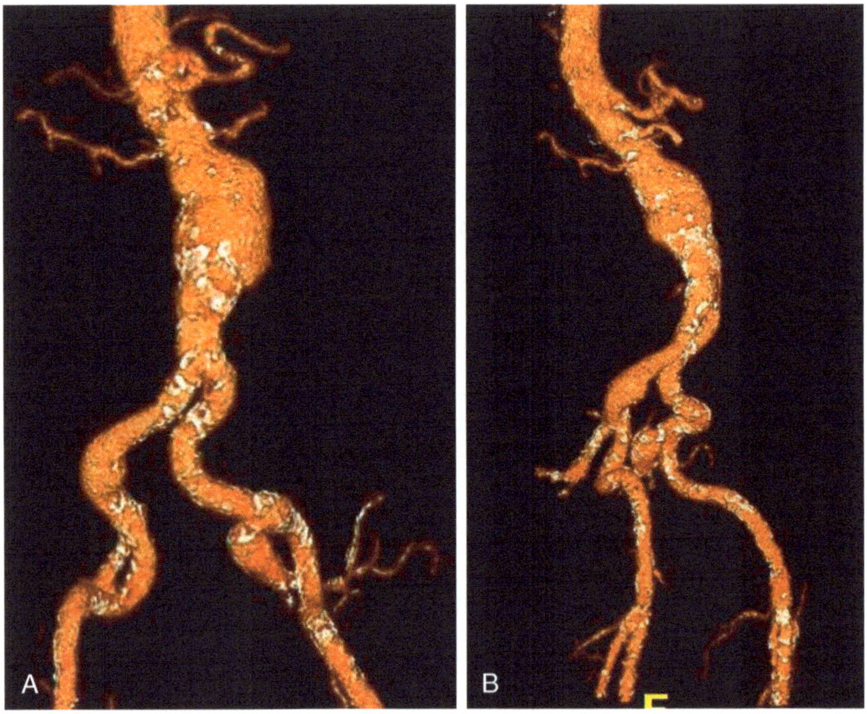

FIG. 10.1 **A, B,** Juxtarenal aortic aneurysm of 74-year-old patient. The patient also had a stenosis of the left renal artery.

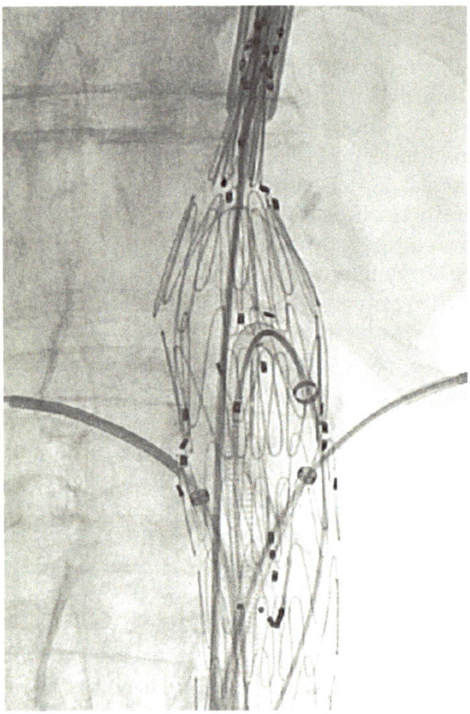

FIG. 10.2 Preloaded fenestrated endograft with extra nitinol wire that passes through the renal fenestrations.

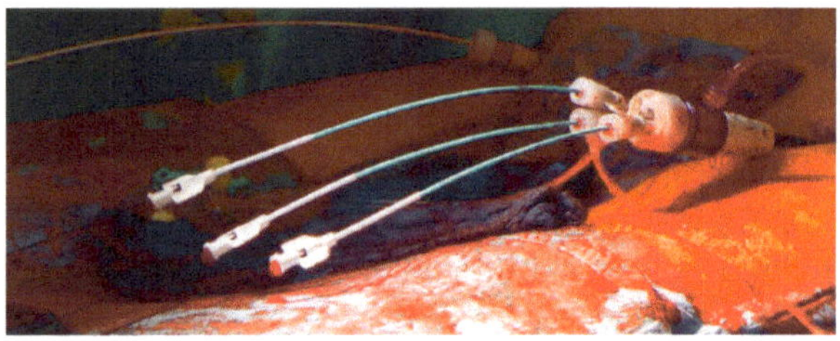

FIG. 10.3 Technique using Prostar XL 10F vascular closure device with triple puncture of the 14F sheath of three 5F sheaths, which will be used for the three aortic side branches, such as the renal arteries and superior mesenteric artery.

Next, 6F Shuttle sheaths (Cook Medical) were advanced into the renal fenestrations over the preloaded wires. The sheath size determines the possible lengths of bridging devices that can be used. For example, with the Advanta/i-Cast V12 (Atrium Medical/Maquet, Hudson, New Hampshire, USA) only the 6-mm-diameter, 22-mm-long device is compatible with the 6F sheath. Consequently, more than one device often must be deployed, an issue that can have detrimental effects on patency. Other centers prefer to

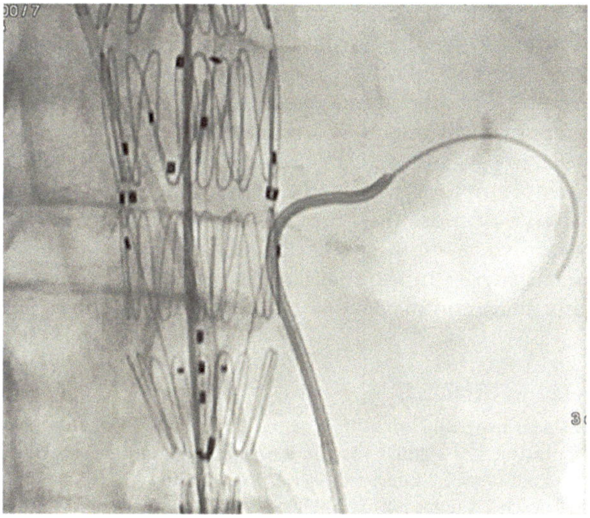

FIG. 10.4 Precannulation of the left renal artery with a Shepherd Hook catheter.

deploy balloon-expandable cobalt-chromium–covered stents, available in longer lengths, with a lower profile possible with the one-layer polytetrafluoroethylene (PTFE) design. However, the use of monolayer PTFE bridging devices for this indication may risk a higher incidence of type III endoleaks, caused by separation of the PTFE coverage from the stent.

Sheath advancement was stopped when the dilators passed through the fenestrations. The Shuttle sheath was then advanced at the level of the lower margin of the fenestration by slowly "benching" and removing the dilator. Then the valve of the Shuttle sheath was punctured with a Cook arterial needle, and a hydrophilic wire (0.035 inch, 180 cm) was passed through this, alongside the preloaded wire. The 4.1F, 100-cm Curly-Q catheter is routinely used for catheterization of the renal arteries. However, any 5F catheter can be used (at least 100 cm long), since the size of the preloaded wire is 0.018 inch. After successful catheterization of the renal arteries, the soft guidewires were replaced with stiffer Rosen wires. The preloaded wire was removed, as were the Shepherd Hook catheters used for the precatheterization of the renal arteries.

The next step was the advancement of the 6F sheaths into the target vessels and catheterization of the SMA from the contralateral groin with one of the two Shepherd Hook catheters used for precatheterization of the renal arteries. Once the catheter was placed through the fenestration and into the SMA, a Rosen wire was parked into the vessel and the prepositioned SMA catheter safely removed.

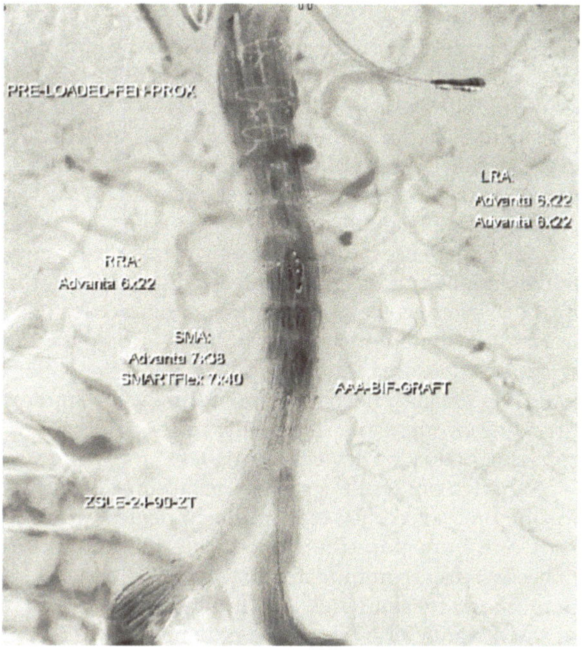

FIG. 10.5 The completed procedure on angiography after placement of the fenestrated endograft, bifurcated device, and ZBIS iliac branch endograft.

A 7F or 8F sheath was then advanced over the Rosen wire and into the SMA. When the SMA and both renal access sheaths were in position, the diameter-reducing ties and the top cap–locking wire were removed. The bare springs were released after moving the top cap to a position above the proximal attachment stent. The selected bridging and relining stent-grafts were safely parked in approximate positions through the fenestrations. The aortic part of the renal stents was flared with the tip of a large angioplasty balloon (10-12 mm).

After angiographic confirmation of patency of all target vessels, the third release ring was removed, releasing the distal attachment and retrieving the top cap. According to the instructions for use, this step should be performed before bridging stent-graft implantation in both renal arteries. However, our experience showed that such an early retrieval of the top cap reduced the space for flaring of the proximal part of the renal bridging stent-graft and could make its visualization during implantation problematic.

Lastly, the proximal component sheath was removed and the distal part (bifurcated graft, iliac branch device [IBD]) implanted in the standard manner (Fig. 10.5). All stent-graft components should be overlapped by at least two stents to avoid late type III endoleak.

DISCUSSION

The standard fenestrated technology has been associated with excellent short-term and midterm clinical outcomes.[2,3] However, several technical issues should be considered. The size of the main sheath (22F to 24F) may cause significant lower-limb ischemia during a 4-hour procedure, and the resulting ischemia-reperfusion syndrome can be fatal.

Our experience is that the new, preloaded fenestrated design leads to a statistically significant reduction in the "sheath-to-target-vessel time" and, accordingly, in the total duration of the procedure. Moreover, the radiation exposure of the surgical team and the patient is also significantly decreased. Interestingly, the amount of iodine contrast was statistically lower in the group receiving preloaded devices.

Although our results suggest some technical benefits for the preloaded FSGs, the modified device carries at least one limitation: the space inside the new introducer system accommodates sheaths of 6F maximum bore for the renal arteries. This limitation excludes use of the Advanta V12, which has a diameter of 0.6 mm and requires a longer length than 22 mm, and is the preferred bridging endograft for renal arteries in our institution. We have solved this problem by routinely molding the Advanta with a larger balloon to fit the anatomy in all patients. We have not experienced any stent-graft dislodgment or fracture. There is risk, however, in patients with large target vessels, so for now we do not employ the preloaded FSG in patients with renal arteries of more than 6 mm diameter. In contrast, 7F sheaths are routinely used for catheterization of both renal arteries in the standard FSGs, which remains an advantage for this device.

REFERENCES

1. Manning BJ, Harris PL, Hartley DE, et al. Preloaded fenestrated stent-grafts for the treatment of juxtarenal aortic aneurysms. *J Endovasc Ther*. 2010;17:456–457.
2. Resch TA, Dias NV, Sobocinski J, et al. Development of off-the-shelf stent grafts for juxtarenal abdominal aortic aneurysms. *Eur J Vasc Endovasc Surg*. 2012;43:655–660.
3. Sobocinski J, d'Utra G, O'Brien N, et al. Off-the-shelf fenestrated endografts: a realistic option for more than 70% of patients with juxtarenal aneurysms. *J Endovasc Ther*. 2012;19:165–172.

CHAPTER 11

Custom-Made Thoracic Endograft

KONSTANTINOS P. DONAS • THEODOSIOS BISDAS • MARTIN AUSTERMANN

Thoracic aortic aneurysms, which affect the unbranched descending aortic segment between the subclavian and celiac arteries with accompanying sufficient landing zones, can be repaired by standard devices. However, more advanced forms of repair are required when the aneurysm involves the aortic arch or extends to the visceral or infrarenal aorta.

These aneurysms can be repaired by entirely endovascular means only if the stent-graft has a branch for each involved target vessel. The branch bridges the gap between the stent-graft and the lumen of the branch artery, maintaining perfusion while excluding the aneurysm.

Cook Medical (Bloomington, Indiana, USA) was the first to provide custom-made devices (CMDs) in a branched configuration. The Cook CMDs were based on the platform of the Zenith endoprosthesis. The proximal sealing zone of the graft consists of one or two sealing stents, with or without an uncovered proximal stent. Proximal barbs are added to the first sealing stent or to the uncovered stent. The length of the covered aorta becomes especially relevant given the risk of spinal cord ischemia in these patients.

The *reducing stent,* which is located distal to the sealing zone, converts the main body into a 16-, 18-, or 22-mm cuff-bearing segment. Based on the aortic lumen, this diameter is planned so that it can accommodate both the main body and the bridging covered stents between the graft side branches and the visceral vessels.

INDICATIONS

- Elective repair of thoracoabdominal aortic aneurysms

PROCEDURE

Case Presentation

A 72-year-old patient presented with a Crawford type II thoracoabdominal aneurysm 7.1 cm in diameter. The patient was a heavy smoker, had severe comorbidities (e.g., chronic obstructive pulmonary disease, previous myocardial infarction), and had a previous abdominal operation for malignancy. The patient chose not to have an open repair. Based on this and the severe comorbidities, we planned a staged procedure to minimize the risk for paraplegia.

First Stage

Deployment of the thoracic device

Chapter 1 describes the percutaneous approach to endovascular aneurysm repair (EVAR). The Prostar system (Abbott Vascular, Redwood City, California, USA) was placed in the common femoral arteries. The operation began with angiography of the renovisceral aorta (Fig. 11.1).

A Lunderquist wire was advanced via transfemoral access and a marker pigtail catheter advanced into the aortic arch (Fig. 11.2). The thoracic device was then deployed in the descending aorta (Fig. 11.3), at least 30 mm above the origin of the celiac trunk.

Second Stage

The second stage of treatment is deployment of the branched device 6 to 8 weeks later.

Step 1. Anesthesia and approach

General anesthesia is used in all patients, and the repairs are performed with a totally percutaneous approach using Prostar XL 10F vascular closure devices (Abbott).

Step 2. Small or stenotic iliac vessels

In patients with small or stenotic iliac vessels, a 10-mm Dacron bypass graft (e.g., B. Braun, USA) between the common iliac and the common femoral artery can be a good option, placed 3 to 4 weeks before the endovascular stent-graft implantation. A staged approach avoids the risk of severe surgical bleeding caused by the advanced heparinization needed for the endovascular repair. In these patients the device is implanted through a small cutdown in the groin.

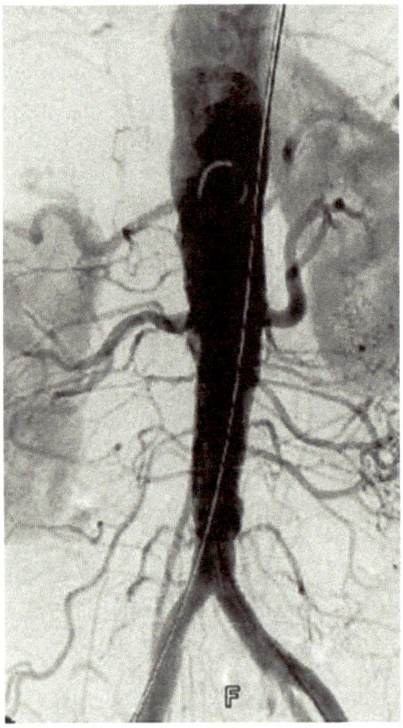

FIG. 11.1 Intraoperative angiography of the renovisceral aorta.

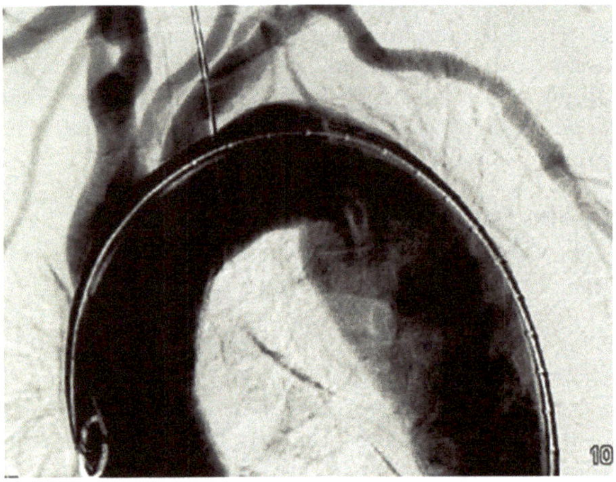

FIG. 11.2 Intraoperative angiography of the aortic arch.

Step 3. Advance of 22F sheath to assess trackability of access vessels

A 22F Check-Flo Introducer sheath (Cook Medical) is provisory, always advanced through the iliac arteries to assess the ease of the branched endograft to pass through the external and common iliac arteries (Fig. 11.4).

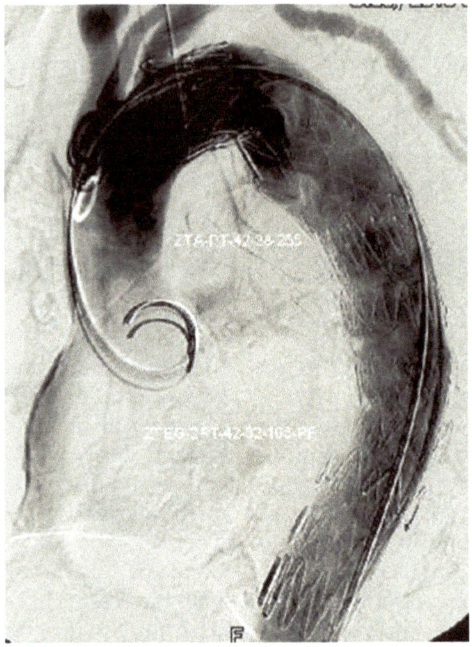

FIG. 11.3 The deployed low-profile tapered Zenith alpha stent-graft of 42-mm and 38-mm diameter for the proximal and the distal edge, respectively, followed by additional Zenith stent-graft tapered with 42-mm and 32-mm proximal and distal diameter, respectively.

Step 4. Release of reducing ties and deployment of device

Withdrawal of the outer sheath is begun after verification of the position and orientation of the branches. As the graft expands, the position of the branches and their relation with the origin of the target vessels will become evident, allowing reorientation of the device if necessary.

After deployment of the distal end of the device and repeat angiography, the spiral stabilizing wire is released and the trigger wire withdrawn. The diameter-reducing ties then are released. After confirmation of graft location, the *black* trigger wire is removed, which releases the graft's proximal attachment. At this phase the distal stent is still secured by the trigger wire. Lastly, the *white* trigger wire is withdrawn and removed to detach the distal end of the endovascular graft (Fig. 11.5).

Techniques to facilitate cannulation of renovisceral vessels

- **Precannulation of visceral vessels**

To maintain proper orientation of the origin of the visceral vessels, we precannulate at least the superior

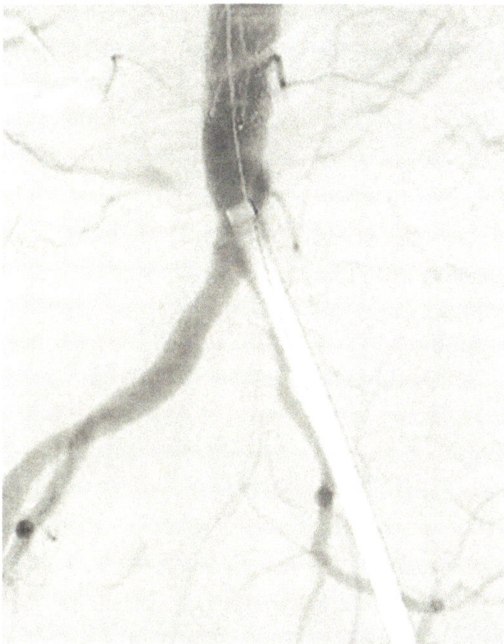

FIG. 11.4 Insertion of the 22F sheath in the common iliac artery. This step is mandatory to ensure the safe advance of the 22F custom-made device.

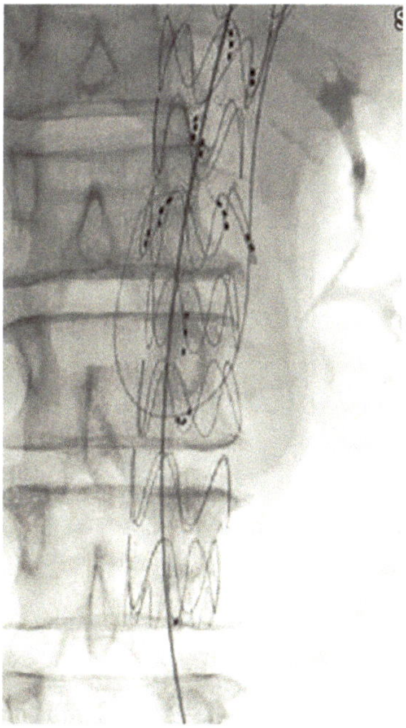

FIG. 11.5 The deployed custom-made device with all markers in the ventral face and at least 20 mm above the origin of the target vessels.

mesenteric artery (SMA) and ideally the two renal arteries before the deployment of the thoracic device. This is accomplished with angulated catheters (e.g., Shepherd Hook, Cobra). After advancing a soft Terumo guidewire in the cannulated target vessels, we fix the wire with a Tru-Boost system.

- **Syngo fusion imaging technique** (Siemens, Munich, Germany)

Step 5. Placement of additional devices

We also advance and deploy the distal component (a bifurcated or tube endograft) to complete the procedure, if necessary, based on the anatomy of the pathologic process.

Step 6. Closure of access in the groin

After closure of the puncture sites of the common femoral artery with the Prostar system, adequate lower-extremity perfusion is assessed, and the groin wounds are closed in layers. This is an important step to minimize the risk for paraplegia and the time of lower-extremity malperfusion.

Step 7. Cannulation of target vessels

After the aortic endograft is in place and the peripheral perfusion restored, the target vessels are cannulated one after the other through the branches, using a 90-cm 8F Shuttle sheath (Cook Medical), combined if necessary with the more flexible dilator of the 110-cm 8F Shuttle sheath. In our experience, the more flexible dilator facilitates advancement of the sheath even in challenging target-vessel anatomies (e.g., angulation or cephalad orientation of renal arteries).

Step 8. Connection of the branches with target vessels

The branches are secured to the target vessels with deployment of stainless steel balloon-expandable covered stents. These bridging endografts are routinely lined with a self-expanding bare-metal stent to provide a more stable transition of the covered stent to the target vessels. When severe angulation of the renal arteries is encountered, additional placement of a flexible self-expanding covered stent will improve the transition of the bridging device in this anatomy. We prefer to start with the cannulation and deployment of the SMA bridging devices because this is the most important branch, where misadventures are life threatening. Fig. 11.6 shows placement of the 7F sheath in the SMA and deployment of the balloon-expandable covered stent.

After revascularization of the SMA, both renal arteries are addressed. Often, the renal arteries of

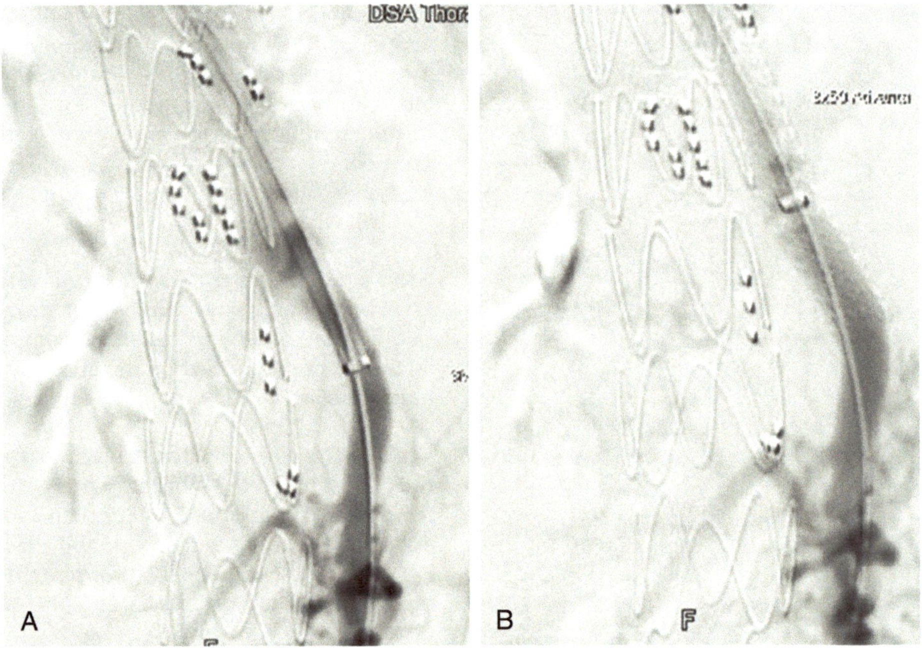

FIG. 11.6 A, B, Cannulation and bridging device placement in the superior mesenteric artery.

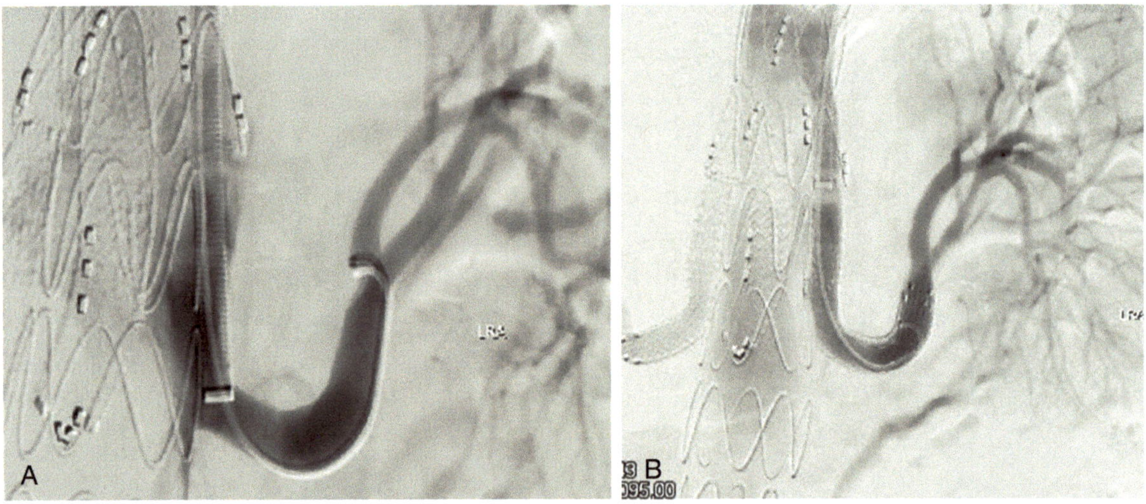

FIG. 11.7 A, B, Superselective angiography of the angulated renal artery after cannulation over the 7F sheath and the combined deployment of the Advanta/i-Cast covered stent proximally and the Viabahn covered stent distally.

thoracoabdominal aneurysms are extremely angulated. Consequently, a rigid bridging device is used proximally and a flexible bridging device distally in the angulated segment of the renal artery. We achieve this hybrid configuration of the bridging device by placement of a balloon-expandable covered device (e.g., Advanta/i-Cast V12, Maquet) proximally and by deployment of a flexible Viabahn device (Gore) distally (Fig. 11.7).

The operator must be careful to note that the Viabahn graft is flexible and can be inadvertently

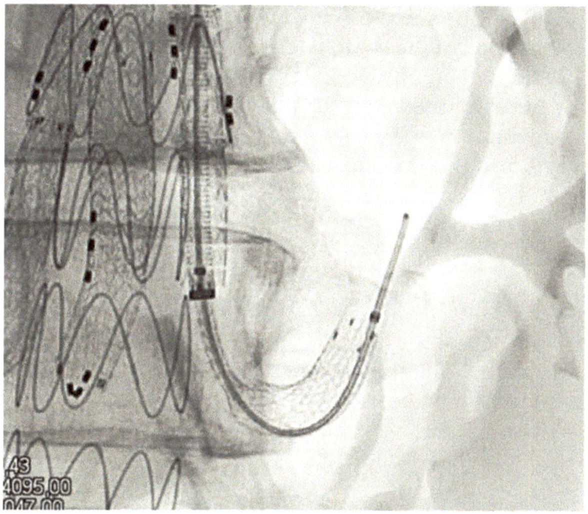

FIG. 11.8 Recommended staged deployment of the Viabahn device with the sheath in position a few centimeters behind the segment of the Viabahn to be deployed.

displaced cranially during the deployment. Therefore, we recommend the *staged release* of the device, with the sheath a few centimeters behind the segment to be deployed, but remaining close to the origin of the branch (Fig. 11.8).

The procedure follows the cannulation and placement of the bridging stent-graft in the celiac trunk. Figs. 11.9 and 11.10 present the next steps of the treatment, addressing the celiac trunk.

Step 9. Completion angiography

The procedure concludes with completion angiography to evaluate the treated segment (Fig. 11.11) and, importantly, the access vessels (Fig. 11.12), to exclude bleeding or peripheral occlusion.

POSTOPERATIVE MANAGEMENT

The following postoperative procedures are important to minimize complications, including delayed paraplegia:

- 48-hour monitoring in an intensive care unit with invasive arterial blood pressure monitoring (mean target, 80-90 mm Hg).
- Selective use of cerebrospinal fluid drainage, limiting its use to patients with clinical signs of postoperative spinal cord ischemia.
- Postoperative imaging to include a control computed tomography (CT) angiography (by glomerular

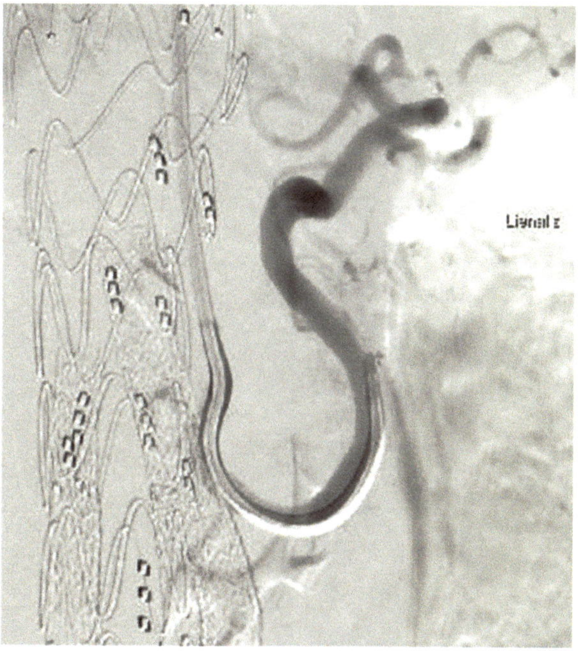

FIG. 11.9 Superselective angiography of the celiac trunk.

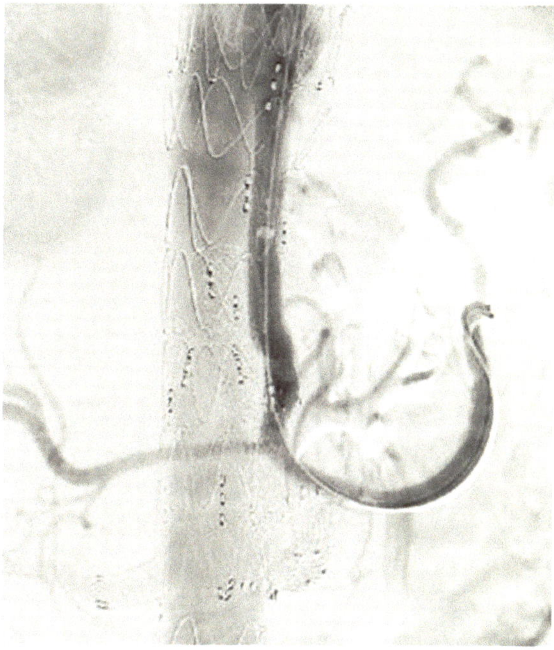

FIG. 11.10 Combined placement of a rigid balloon-expandable covered stent proximally and a flexible self-expanding covered stent distally.

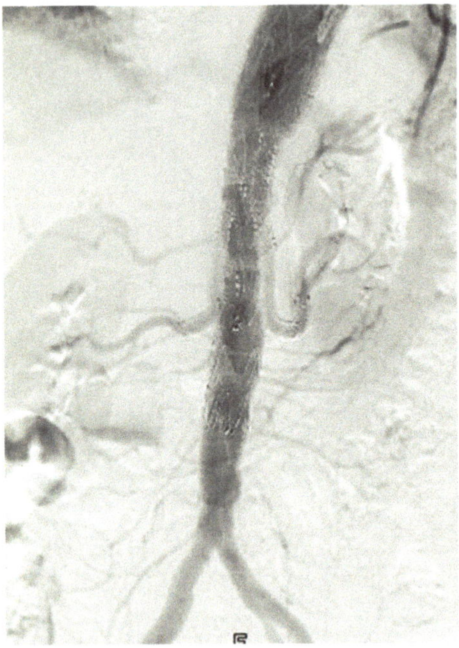

FIG. 11.11 Completion angiography highlighting patent renovisceral vessels and exclusion of the aneurysm.

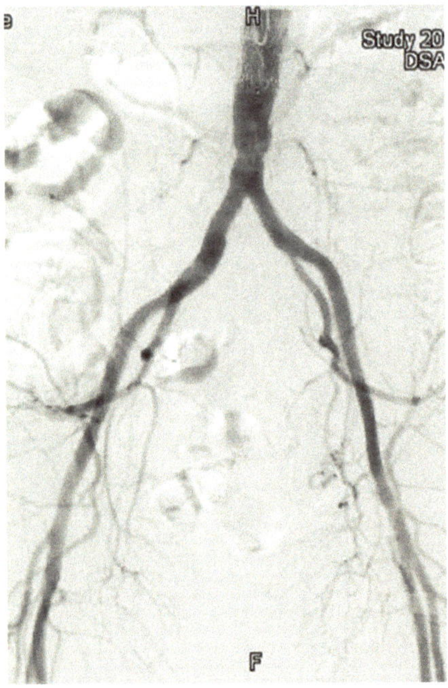

FIG. 11.12 Evaluation of the perfusion of the iliac and common femoral arteries on completion angiography.

filtration rate >60 mL/min/1.73 m^2) and x-ray imaging of the stent. Follow-up imaging consists of CT angiography and x-ray images at 12 months and annually thereafter. In patients with renal impairment, non-contrast-enhanced CT scans and duplex ultrasound imaging can be performed to assess aneurysm size and patency of the target vessels, respectively.

LIMITATIONS OF CUSTOM-MADE ENDOGRAFT

The main limitation for the use of CMDs is the time required for manufacturing, usually at least 4 weeks, with the associated risk for aneurysm rupture, especially with large diameters.

LITERATURE REVIEW

Troisi et al.[1] published the Münster, Germany, experience with branched devices for the treatment of pararenal and thoracoabdominal aortic aneurysms in 2011. Between January 2001 and May 2010, 107 consecutive high-risk patients (97 men; mean age, 73 years; range, 50-86) were treated with a CMD Zenith endograft. The 30-day mortality rate was 1.9%. During follow-up (mean, 25 months; range, 1-94), 34 secondary procedures were performed in 28 patients (26.2%). The mean interval between the primary and secondary procedures was 12.9 months (range, 1-68). In 26 (76.5%) of 34 cases, a secondary endovascular procedure was performed; in the remaining eight cases (23.5%), the complication was treated surgically. Type III endoleak was the most common cause for reintervention during follow-up. Estimated 3-year survival was 77%, and the 3-year rate for freedom from any device-related secondary procedure was 75.5%.

The authors found that the incidence of early and late complications requiring a secondary procedure after treatment with fenestrated or branched devices was not negligible. Accurate preoperative planning, the advent of new materials and techniques, and strict follow-up could be the key factors in improving the results of fenestrated or branched stent-graft interventions and reducing the rate of secondary procedures.

Also in 2011, Austermann et al.[2] reported lessons learned after review of the causes leading to secondary procedures. They proposed several modifications to the technique to improve the results of this approach for complex aortic aneurysm repair.

REFERENCES

1. Troisi N, Donas KP, Austermann M, et al. Secondary procedures after aortic aneurysm repair with fenestrated and branched endografts. *J Endovasc Ther*. 2011;18(2):146–153.
2. Austermann M, Donas KP, Panuccio G, et al. Pararenal and thoracoabdominal aortic aneurysm repair with fenestrated and branched endografts: lessons learned and future directions. *J Endovasc Ther*. 2011;18(2):157–160.

CHAPTER 12

Off-the-Shelf Multibranched Endograft

KONSTANTINOS P. DONAS • THEODOSIOS BISDAS • MARTIN AUSTERMANN

To overcome the delay of custom manufacturing and to offer an off-the-shelf solution for use in urgent conditions, a new device was designed, the t-branch thoracic endograft. This off-the-shelf device has an introduction delivery system that consists of a 22-French (22F) Flexor introducer sheath (7.3-mm inner diameter [ID] and 8.5-mm outer diameter [OD]) and a Captor hemostatic valve (Cook Medical, Bloomington, Indiana, USA). The system has a fixed proximal diameter of 34 mm and a distal diameter of 18 mm. Cook Medical provides a universal distal body at four different sizes, with proximal diameter (D) always 22 mm; lengths (L) of 81, 98, 115, and 132 mm; and 20F delivery system (Fig. 12.1).

The device was created to overcome the limitations of the custom-made multibranched endograft. Consequently, symptomatic and ruptured thoracoabdominal aortic aneurysms (TAAAs) can now be treated with this device.

ANATOMIC REQUIREMENTS

1. **Proximal to aneurysm.** The device requires a 25-mm-long segment of nonaneurysmal thoracic aorta for proximal fixation, with an angle of less than 90 degrees relative to the long axis of the aneurysm, length of at least 25 mm, and diameter measured *outer wall to outer wall* no greater than 30 mm and no less than 24 mm. Alternatively, the device may be attached to a preexisting thoracic endovascular graft.
2. **Visceral vessel anatomy**
   a. Four indispensable arteries
   b. Aortic diameter greater than 25 mm at the region of the branches
   c. Target vessel accessible from antegrade approach
   d. Celiac and superior mesenteric artery (SMA) 6 to 10 mm in diameter
   e. Renal arteries 4 to 8 mm in diameter
   f. Distance between the cuff and the corresponding arterial orifice less than 50 mm
   g. The line between the cuff and the arterial orifice, as projected onto the vessel wall, deviates no more than 45 degrees from the long axis of the aorta.
3. **Access**
   a. Adequate iliac/femoral access compatible with a 22F (8.5-mm OD) delivery system
   b. Brachial, axillary, or subclavian access vessel size compatible with the delivery profile of a 10F or 12F introducer sheath (3.3- or 4-mm OD).

INDICATIONS

- Elective pararenal or thoracoabdominal aneurysms
- Symptomatic or ruptured pararenal or thoracoabdominal aneurysms

PROCEDURE

Case Presentation

A 72-year-old male patient presented with a 6.8-cm type V TAAA (Fig. 12.2), based on the Crawford Classification modified by Safi and Miller.[1] The patient had a previous myocardial infarction and coronary stent placement, chronic obstructive pulmonary disease (GOLD III), arterial hypertension, and diabetes mellitus type 2.

Procedural Steps

Step 1. Anesthesia and approach

All patients undergo general anesthesia and a totally percutaneous approach using the Prostar XL 10F vascular closure device (Abbott Vascular, Redwood City, California, USA).

Importance of Activated Clotting Time (ACT) Measurement. Heparin is administered at a dose of 100 IU/kg body weight, aiming for an ACT of at least 250 seconds. ACT measurements should be performed every 30 minutes.

Step 2. Small or stenotic iliac vessels

In elective, asymptomatic patients with small or stenotic iliac vessels, a 10-mm Dacron bypass graft (e.g., B. Braun, USA) can be implanted between the common iliac and the common femoral artery 3 to 4 weeks before planned aneurysm repair. A two-stage approach

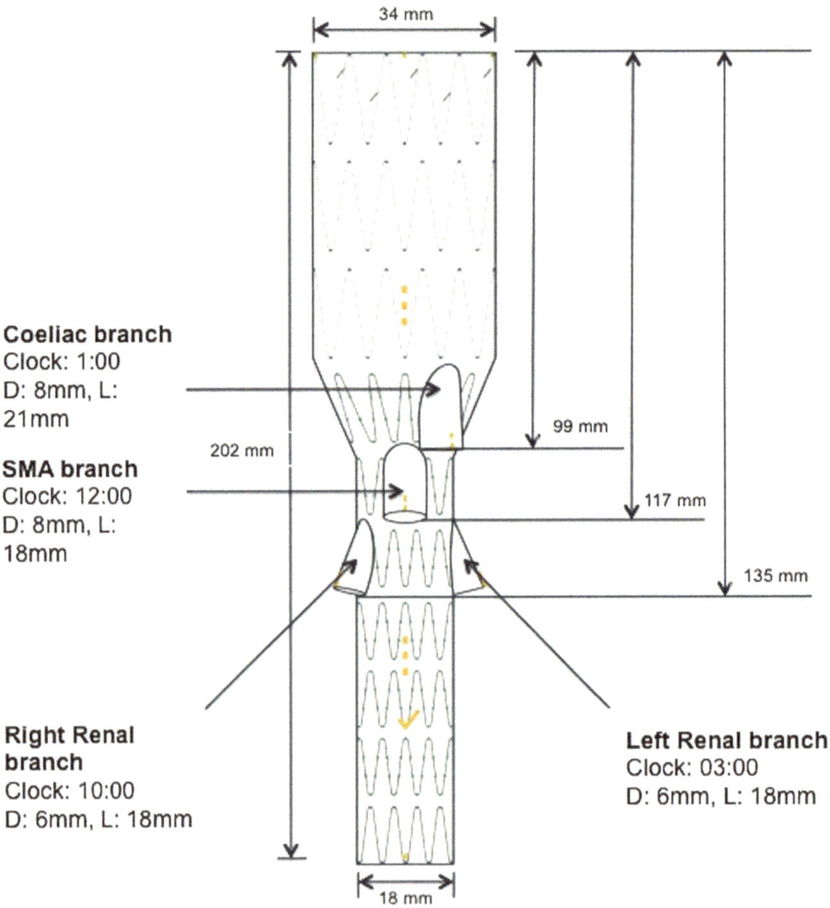

FIG. 12.1 Features of the t-branch device. *SMA*, Superior mesenteric artery; *coeliac*, celiac. (From Bisdas T, Donas KP, Bosiers MJ, et al. Custom-made versus off-the-shelf multibranched endografts for endovascular repair of thoracoabdominal aortic aneurysms. J Vasc Surg 2014;60(5):1188.)

avoids severe surgical bleeding from the high-dose heparinization needed for the endovascular repair. In these patients the device is implanted through a small cutdown in the groin.

Step 3. Advancement of 22F sheath to assess trackability of access vessels

A 22F Check-Flo Introducer sheath (Cook Medical) is always advanced through the iliac arteries to assess the ability of the branched endograft to pass through the external and common iliac arteries (Fig. 12.3).

If this maneuver is successful, the procedure continues with SMA precannulation with a Shepherd Hook catheter (Boston Scientific, Natick, Massachusetts, USA) placed in the contralateral groin. Alternatively, Syngo fusion imaging (Siemens, Munich, Germany) can be used to accurately identify the target vessels.

In patients with TAAA involving the arch or descending aorta, the proximal thoracic component can be implanted in a staged approach. In this case, and if the patient is asymptomatic, we prefer a staged procedure with an interval of at least 6 to 8 weeks between the implantation of the thoracic device and the t-branch.

Step 4. Advancement of device at least 10 to 20 mm above orifice of respective target vessel

The t-branch is advanced and deployed by withdrawing the outer sheath so that the branches are located at least 10 to 20 mm above the orifice of each respective target vessel, previously marked with the catheter placed into the involved target vessels.

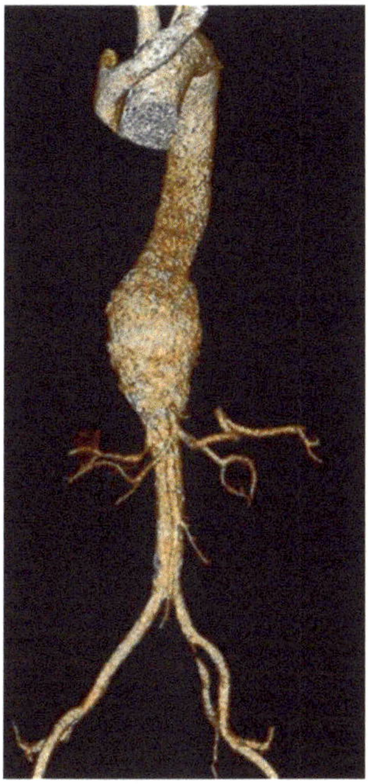

FIG. 12.2 A 6.8-cm thoracoabdominal aortic aneurysm extending from the distal thoracic aorta, including the celiac and superior mesenteric origins, but terminating proximal to the renal arteries.

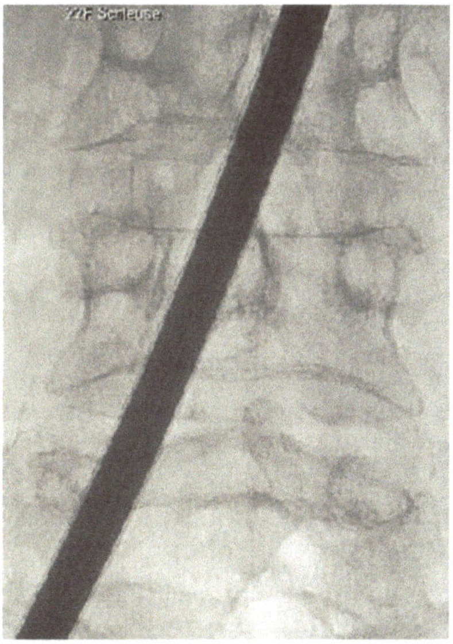

FIG. 12.3 The pre–thoracic stent-graft deployment "testing" of the iliac artery's ability to advance a 22F sheath in the common iliac artery. If successful, the t-branch will be prepared for placement. Image shows the insertion of the 22F sheath in the common iliac artery.

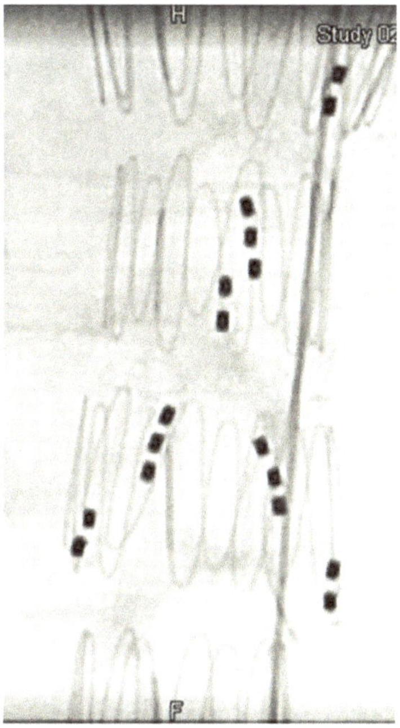

FIG. 12.4 The fully deployed t-branch device.

Step 5. Release of reducing ties and deployment of device

The reducing ties are released, and the aortic endograft repair is completed with the implantation of the distal component (tube or bifurcated device). All sheaths are removed, with suture closure of femoral arterial puncture sites. We *completely* deploy the t-branch before the transaxillary delivery of the bridging endografts to avoid a long occlusion time of the limbs and the hypogastric arteries. This should minimize the risk for paraplegia. Fig. 12.4 shows the deployed t-branch with all markers in the ventral face of the device.

Step 6. Cannulation of target vessels

After the aortic endografts are in place and the femoral arteries are closed, the target vessels are cannulated one after the other through the branches, using a 90-cm 8F Shuttle sheath, combined, however, with the more flexible dilator of the 110-cm 7F Shuttle sheath (Cook Medical). In our experience, the more flexible dilator facilitates the advancement of the sheath in challenging target-vessel anatomies (e.g., angulation or cephalic orientation of renal arteries).

Step 7. Connection of the branches with target vessels

The branches are sealed to the target vessels using stainless steel balloon-expandable covered stents. The bridging

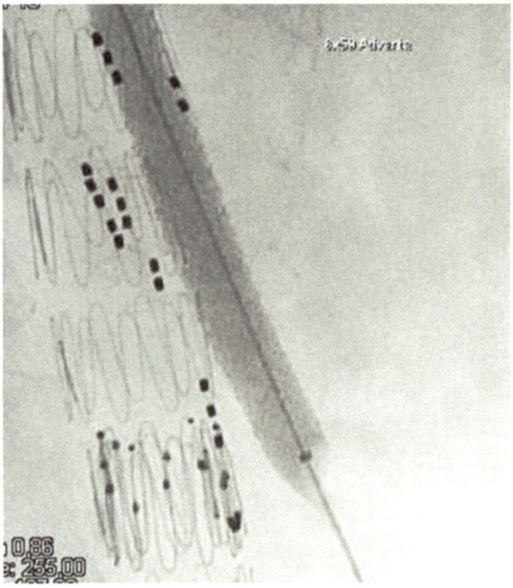

FIG. 12.5 Balloon-expandable covered stent (Advanta/i-Cast V12; 8 × 59 mm) in the superior mesenteric artery.

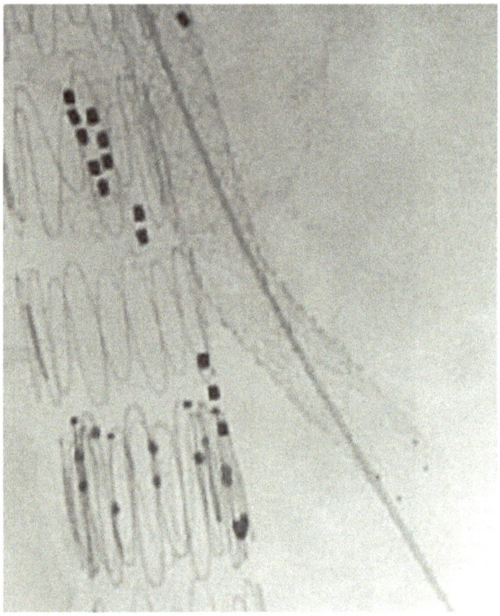

FIG. 12.6 Completed deployment, with the Advanta/i-Cast bridging device lined with a bare-metal stent in the superior mesenteric artery.

endograft is routinely lined with a self-expanding bare-metal stent to provide a more gradual and stable transition of the covered stent to the native artery. The additional stent is particularly important in cases of severe angulation of the renal arteries, where the flexible self-expanding covered stent is necessary for a smooth transition.

Deployment of the SMA bridging devices is performed first, since this is the most important target vessel. Fig. 12.5 shows the deployed bridging device, a balloon-expandable stainless steel covered stent in the SMA.

The device will be lined by placement of an additional nitinol bare-metal stent. Fig. 12.6 shows the lined Advanta/i-Cast graft.

After revascularization of the SMA, both renal arteries are addressed. Fig. 12.7 shows the superselective angiogram after cannulation of the right renal artery over the 7F sheath.

Each renal artery is treated in a manner similar to that described for the SMA, using balloon-expandable covered stents (Fig. 12.8).

As described, we recommend additional placement of a flexible nitinol stent to improve the transition of the rigid Advanta/i-Cast in these severe angulations (Fig. 12.9). The additional stent improves the transition and comformability of the bridging device when challenging renal artery anatomy is encountered.

The final angiography confirms a patent renal artery without evidence of peripheral embolization or dissection (Fig. 12.10).

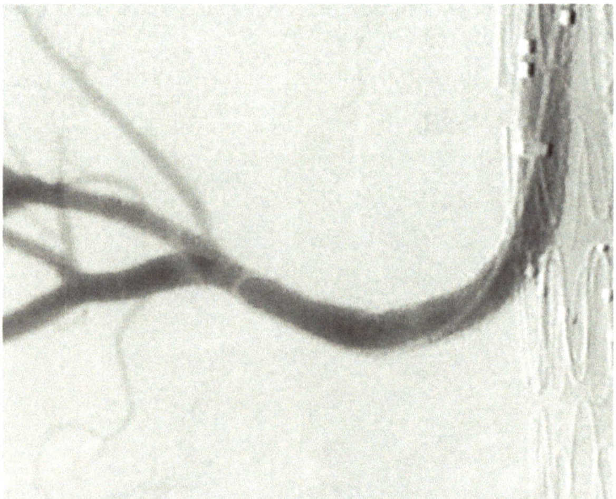

FIG. 12.7 Superselective angiography after successful placement of the 7F sheath in the right renal artery.

Angiography of the aneurysm sac through the still-open branch of the celiac artery branch can be useful to evaluate possible intercostal or lumbar arteries that might communicate with the anterior spinal artery. Should such relevant arteries be observed, the branch of the celiac trunk should remain open, with connection to the target vessel in a third procedure 6 to 8 weeks later.

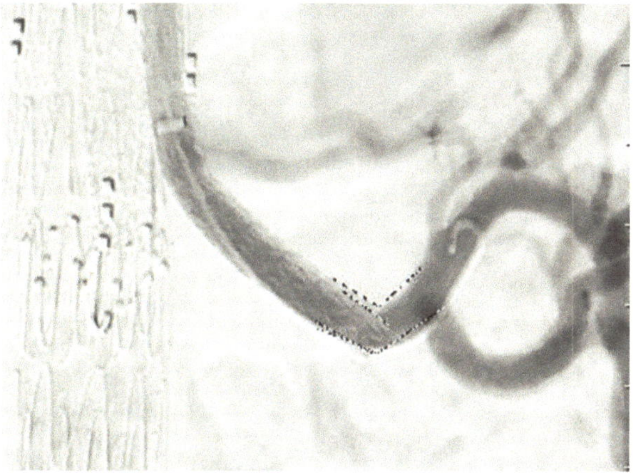

FIG. 12.8 Placement of the bridging device in the left renal artery; in this case highlighting severe angulation of the renal artery. Placement of a rigid stainless steel bridging device in an upward-oriented renal artery requires additional intervention in the form of a bare-metal stent to achieve a smooth transition without kinking.

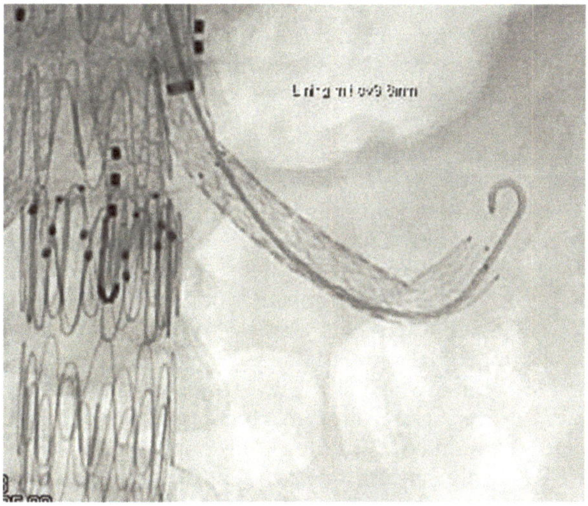

FIG. 12.9 The lined rigid balloon-expandable covered stent, with the flexible nitinol stent creating a funnel at the distal edge of the bridging device.

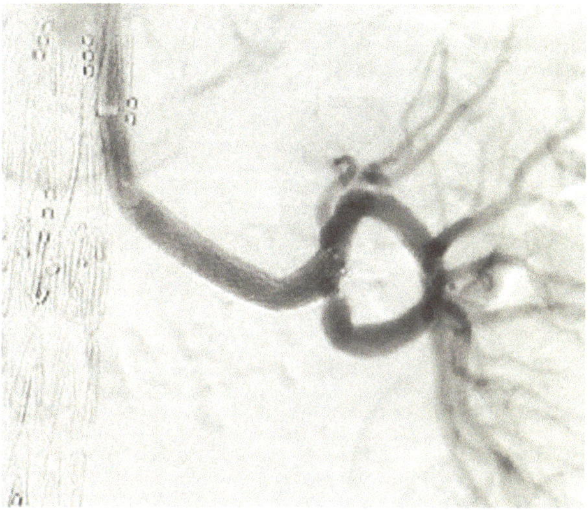

FIG. 12.10 Superselective angiography of the renal artery after placement of the bridging devices.

If no such communication is seen, a balloon-expandable covered stent is placed in the celiac trunk branch, with an additional self-expanding bare-metal stent to complete the repair.

Step 8. Completion angiography

At the end of the procedure, completion angiography is performed to confirm patency of the target vessels and bridging devices. Fig. 12.11 shows the final result, with successful exclusion of the type V TAAA.

Step 9. Evaluation of perfusion of hypogastric arteries

One of the most crucial parameters to ensure the success of the treatment is the absence of a persistent postoperative neurologic deficit. We emphasize again the importance of the rapid removal of all sheaths and catheters in the iliac arteries after deployment of the stent-graft, to minimize the duration of ischemia to the pelvis and, through collaterals, to the spinal cord itself.

In this context, we highlight the importance of patent hypogastric arteries without significant stenosis. Fig. 12.12 shows a high-grade stenosis of the left hypogastric artery. In this case the hypogastric artery was cannulated from the upper extremity, and a balloon-expandable bare-metal stent (e.g., Dynamic Renal, Biotronik, Berlin, Germany) 5 mm in diameter and 18 mm in length was successfully deployed (Fig. 12.13).

Summary

We perform three intraoperative techniques to minimize the risk for postoperative paraplegia:

1. Angiography of the aneurysm sac through the still-open branch of the celiac artery, to identify relevant intercostal or lumbar arteries that might communicate with the anterior spinal artery. In this case the branch of the celiac trunk will be left open and connected to the target vessel at a third procedure 6 to 8 weeks later.

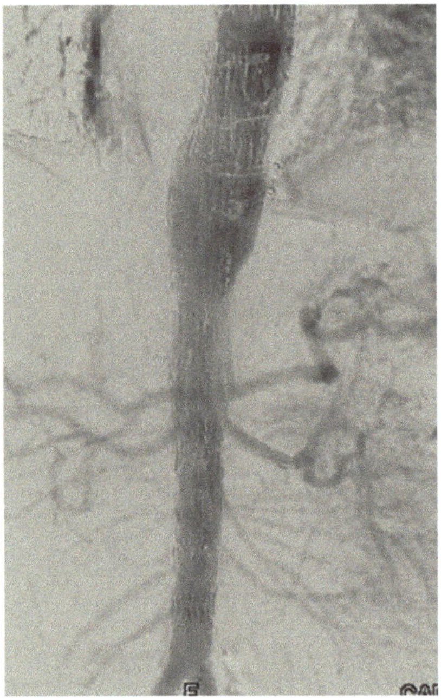

FIG. 12.11 Successful exclusion of the type V thoracoabdominal aortic aneurysm (visceral aneurysm) by the t-branch device.

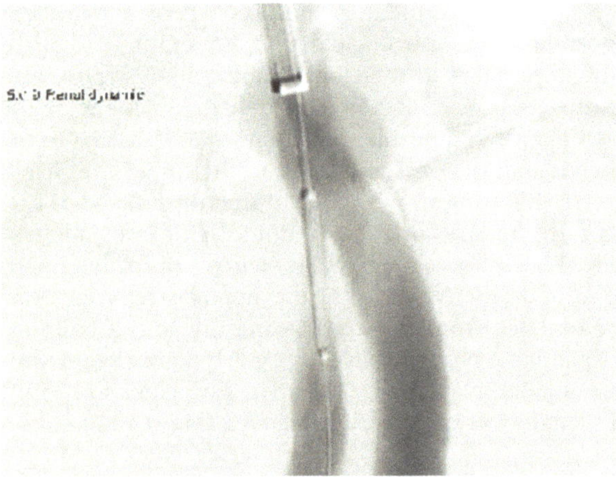

FIG. 12.12 High-grade stenosis of left hypogastric artery.

2. Closure of the common femoral arterial access sites after the deployment of the t-branch. All layers of the groin sites are closed, including the skin before cannulation of the target vessels and deployment of the bridging devices from the upper extremity.
3. Evaluation of hypogastric artery perfusion, with remediation of moderate- or high-grade stenosis with balloon-expandable stents, to optimize perfusion and reduce the risk of spinal cord ischemia.

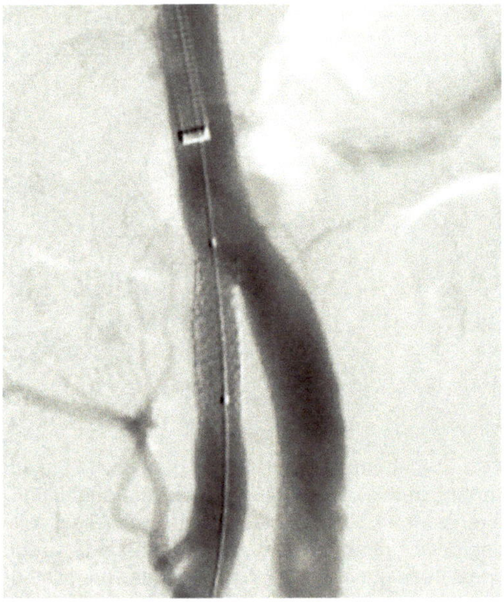

FIG. 12.13 Final angiographic result of repair of hypogastric artery in Fig. 12.12, with patent vessel and no evidence of residual stenosis.

POSTOPERATIVE MANAGEMENT

- 48-hour monitoring in an intensive care unit with invasive arterial blood pressure monitoring to keep the mean pressure between 80 and 90 mm Hg.
- Selective use of cerebrospinal fluid drainage, limiting its use to patients with clinical signs of postoperative spinal cord ischemia.
- Postoperative imaging with computed tomography (CT) angiography (when glomerular filtration rate >60 mL/min/1.73 m^2) and x-ray imaging of the stent. Follow-up imaging includes CT angiography and x-ray images at 12 months and annually thereafter. In patients with renal impairment, non-contrast-enhanced CT scan and duplex ultrasound imaging can be performed to assess the changes in aneurysm size, presence of endoleaks, and patency of the target vessels.

LIMITATIONS OF OFF-THE-SHELF ENDOGRAFT

The main anatomic limitations for further application of the t-branch device are as follows:

- Distance between the celiac trunk and the most caudal renal artery greater than 56 mm

- Insufficient aortic diameter (<25 mm) at the level of the visceral arteries
- Upward orientation of one or both renal arteries
- Inadequate (>40 mm) diameter of the proximal landing zone
- A distance of less than 67 mm between the most caudal renal artery and the aortic bifurcation, as may be encountered in patients with previous open repair of the abdominal aorta with a bifurcated graft

LITERATURE REVIEW

Bosiers et al.[2] first reported the clinical application of the t-branch device in 15 patients with TAAA. Use of the t-branch device proved to be feasible and safe, with encouraging early clinical and radiologic outcomes. Every target vessel was successfully connected, with 100% early branch patency and no mortality.

Bisdas et al.[3] compared the efficacy of the first off-the-shelf multibranched endograft (t-branch) for endovascular aneurysm repair (EVAR) with the traditional custom-made device (CMD). Technically and clinically, the outcomes were similar. Compared with the t-branch device, however, the CMD was associated with better early performance, although not statistically significant. The 6-month freedom-from-reintervention rate was 100% and 90% for the t-branch and CMD, respectively.

There remain a number of anatomic obstacles that contraindicate the suitability of the t-branch device or require the performance of adjuvant procedures such as carotid-subclavian bypass or additional proximal thoracic endograft placement. These adjunctive procedures can be accompanied by additional morbidity. Regarding the anatomic contraindications for use of the t-branch device, we observed an inadequate distance (>56 mm) between the celiac trunk and the most caudal renal artery and an insufficient diameter (<25 mm) at the level of the visceral arteries as the reasons for exclusion of patients in 60% and 33% of cases, respectively.

In summary, use of the t-branch device allows urgent treatment of patients with symptomatic TAAA and those with impending rupture. Cannulation of the target vessels through the branches of the device makes the procedure safe.

Further, the widespread application of a CMD is not relevant to the off-the shelf endograft for several reasons. First, the branches of custom-made endografts are usually placed at the most optimal position above the target vessels, facilitating their catheterization. Besides, in TAAAs with a proximal landing zone greater than 32 mm in diameter, the CMD can be ordered with a proximal diameter of 38 mm. In contrast, the t-branch device, having a fixed diameter of 34 mm, requires a proximal extension with an additional thoracic endograft, which can be a risk for postoperative paraplegia. Moreover, in patients with suprarenal aneurysms, the custom-made endograft can be manufactured with two stents at the proximal part, in contrast to the fixed three stents of the t-branch device, thereby reducing the risk for postoperative paraplegia.

REFERENCES

1. Safi HJ, Miller 3rd CC. Spinal cord protection in descending thoracic and thoracoabdominal aortic repair. *Ann Thorac Surg*. 1999;67:1937–1939.
2. Bosiers M, Bisdas T, Donas KP, et al. Early clinical experience with the first commercially available off-the-shelf multibranched endograft in the treatment of thoracoabdominal aortic aneurysms. *J Endovasc Ther*. 2013;20:719–725.
3. Bisdas T, Donas KP, Bosiers MJ, et al. Custom-made versus off-the-shelf multibranched endografts for endovascular repair of thoracoabdominal aortic aneurysms. *J Vasc Surg*. 2014;60(5):1188.

CHAPTER 13

Sandwich Endovascular Technique

KONSTANTINOS P. DONAS • THEODOSIOS BISDAS

The sandwich endovascular technique is an option for the total endovascular treatment of thoracoabdominal aortic aneurysms (TAAAs). The technique consists of three major steps: (1) deployment of a thoracic stent-graft in a healthy, nonaneurysmal aortic segment of the thoracic aorta; (2) placement of long, self-expanding covered stents in the involved renovisceral vessels; and (3) deployment of abdominal tube endografts between the long, covered stents and the abdominal aorta. This creates the following configuration, from outer to inner side: thoracic device, self-expanding covered stents running from the aortic side branches to the proximal level of the thoracic device (chimney grafts) or to the distal abdominal aorta (periscopes), and lastly, abdominal tube endografts to cover the distal portion of the aneurysm in the abdominal aorta. The three "layers" of endovascular devices in the thoracoabdominal aorta (thoracic endograft > chimney or periscope grafts > abdominal tubes) create the term *sandwich technique*, or *wrap technique*.

INDICATIONS

- Elective repair of TAAAs
- Symptomatic or ruptured TAAAs
- Type Ia endoleaks after endovascular aortic repair

PROCEDURE

Case Presentation

The patient presented with a contained, ruptured aneurysm from a type Ia endoleak after fenestrated endovascular repair; originally performed in 2005 using a device with two fenestrations. In 2009 the patient underwent reintervention with placement of balloon-expandable covered stents in both renal arteries as a result of fracture of the right balloon-expandable bare-metal stent, which was primarily deployed. At this time the patient had an endoleak from the right renal artery, with significant expansion of the aneurysm sac. Seven years later, the patient presented with a contained rupture. Fig. 13.1 shows the new onset of type Ia endoleak based on computed tomography angiography (CTA).

The cause for the type Ia endoleak was fracture at the origin of the fenestrations (Fig. 13.2).

Procedural Steps

1. Exposure of left axillary artery

The axillary artery was exposed through an incision in the deltopectoral groove. The pectoralis major muscle was divided in the direction of its fibers, as was the pectoralis minor muscle from its the insertion on the coracoid process.

2. Percutaneous transfemoral access

Percutaneous transfemoral access was achieved, using the Prostar XL device (Abbott) in a "preclose" technique. Stiff guidewires were advanced into the aorta, as in standard thoracic endovascular aortic repair (TEVAR).

3. Deployment of thoracic endograft

Thoracic endografts are chosen, as available at the center, including a stainless steel or nitinol endoskeleton. In this case the lower end of the graft was positioned as close as possible to the origin of the celiac trunk (Fig. 13.3).

4. Placement of infrarenal aortic stent-graft

This step involves placement of a bifurcated infrarenal aortic stent graft, cannulation of the contralateral iliac limb, and deployment of the iliac graft. In the event of a distal nonaneurysmal landing zone more than 2 cm in length, deployment of an aortic tube is preferred.

In this case the infrarenal aortic stent-graft is the fenestrated endograft.

5. Cannulation of renovisceral vessels

Cannulation of Visceral Arteries. Puncture of the left axillary artery is performed, or bilateral transbrachial cannulation from the upper extremities (antecubital level). After the double puncture of the left axillary artery, with 1 to 2 cm between the punctures, two short 5-French (5F) sheaths are advanced (Fig. 13.4).

The next step is the placement of a pigtail catheter over a soft Terumo wire (Terumo Medical, Somerset, New Jersey, USA) in the renovisceral aorta. After

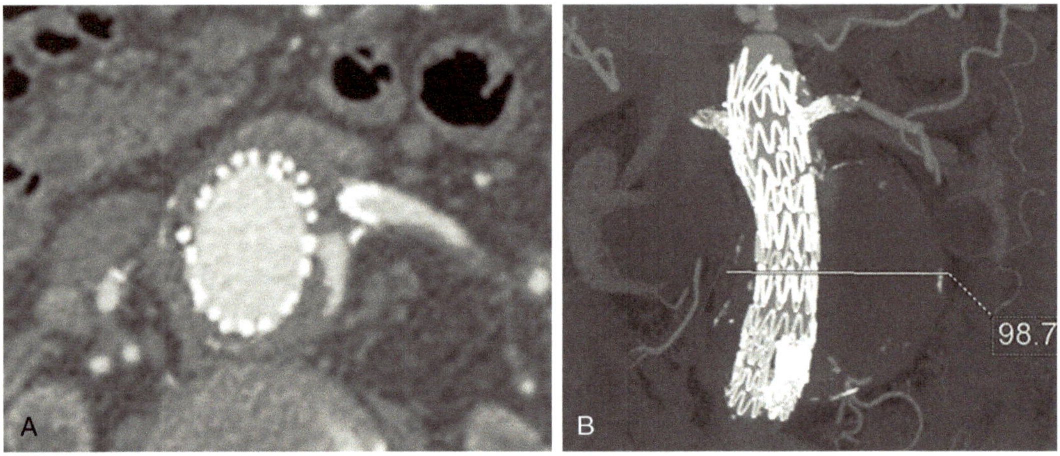

FIG. 13.1 A, B, New onset of type Ia endoleak with contained rupture after fenestrated endograft placement 11 years earlier.

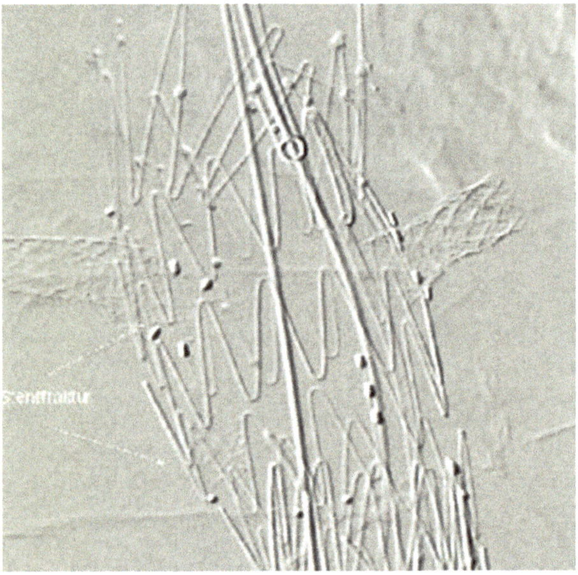

FIG. 13.2 Fenestrated endograft with evidence of fracture of the fenestration stents.

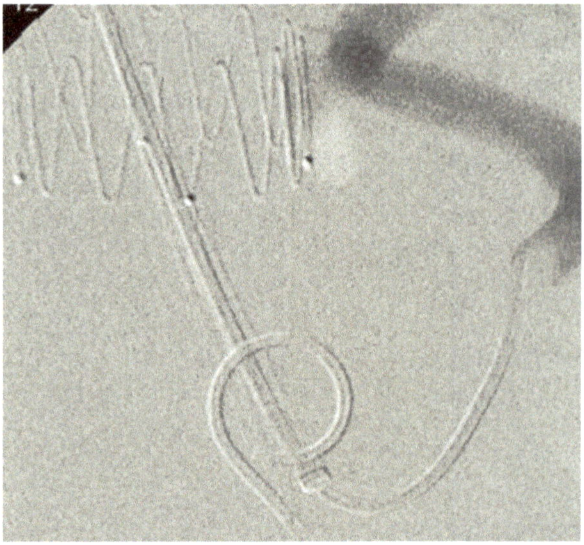

FIG. 13.3 Caudal edge of the deployed thoracic stent-graft above origin of the celiac artery.

exchange with a stiff wire, a long 7F Shuttle sheath (Cook Medical) is advanced into the renovisceral aorta.

As a second option, bilateral exposure of the brachial artery may be performed. After puncture or cutdown of the brachial artery and placement of a short 4F or 5F sheath using the Seldinger technique, a soft Terumo wire is advanced in the ascending aorta. In addition, a pigtail catheter is advanced into the aortic arch. After positioning of the curved tip of the catheter in the side of the descending aorta, a sudden advance of the guidewire with simultaneous removal of the pigtail catheter backward will bring the catheter into the renovisceral segment. The same technique is performed for the right brachial artery. After advance of a stiff wire in the renovisceral segment, the pigtail catheter will be removed and a 8F Shuttle sheath (Cook Medical) will be placed above the visceral arteries.

The cannulation of the visceral arteries is performed with angled-tip catheters such as the Vertebral or the M.P.A. Additionally, the soft Terumo wire is advanced in the renal artery, followed by the catheter. After removal

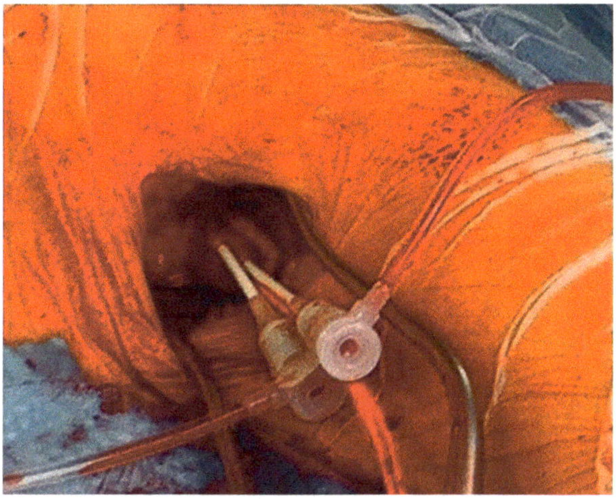

FIG. 13.4 Double-puncture technique of the axillary artery.

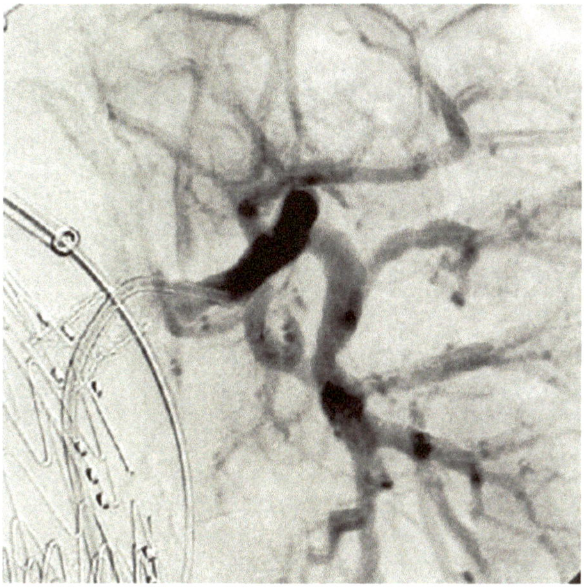

FIG. 13.5 Superselective angiogram of the left renal artery after successful cannulation, excluding iatrogenic dissection or other injury during cannulation.

of the wire and superselective angiography of the renal artery, the stiff wire with curved-tip Rosen wire (Cook Medical) is placed in the visceral arteries. The sheaths are then advanced at least 15 mm into the visceral arteries.

Transfemoral Cannulation of Renal Arteries from Right and Left Groin. A Vertebral or Shepherd Hook catheter can be used to introduce a soft Terumo wire into the renal arteries first. Fig. 13.5 depicts a superselective angiogram of the left renal artery after successful cannulation, excluding iatrogenic dissection or other injury during cannulation.

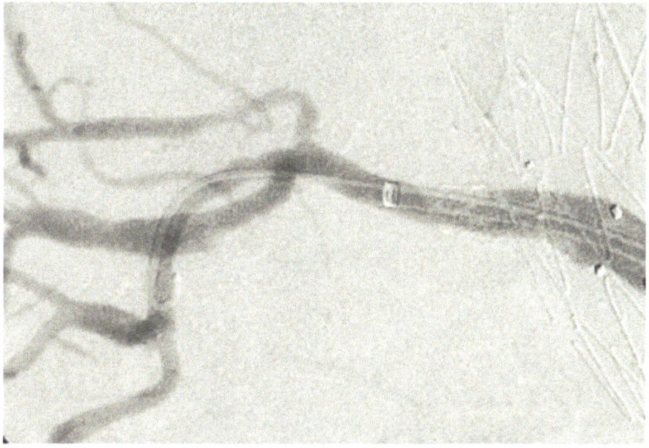

FIG. 13.6 Insertion of the 8F sheath over an atraumatic curved-tip (Rosen) wire into the right renal artery.

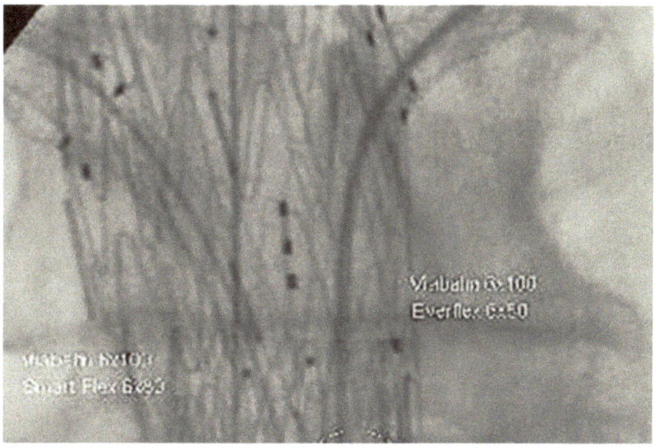

FIG. 13.7 Transfemoral placement of Viabahn self-expanding covered stents in the renal arteries, additionally lined by deployment of self-expanding bare-metal stents (ev3 Everflex Protege).

After exchange for a stiff, 0.035-inch Rosen wire, a long 8F sheath was introduced transfemorally into the renal artery and superselective angiography performed (Fig. 13.6).

The Viabahn grafts were then placed into the renal arteries in a caudally facing configuration as periscopes. To improve the radial force of the Viabahn grafts, additional bare-metal stents can be deployed. In this case we deployed a self-expanding bare-metal stent (ev3 Protege, Medtronic) (Fig 13.7).

6. *Deployment of abdominal tube endografts*

The last step of the procedure consists of deployment of the aortic stent grafts, oversized by about 30%.

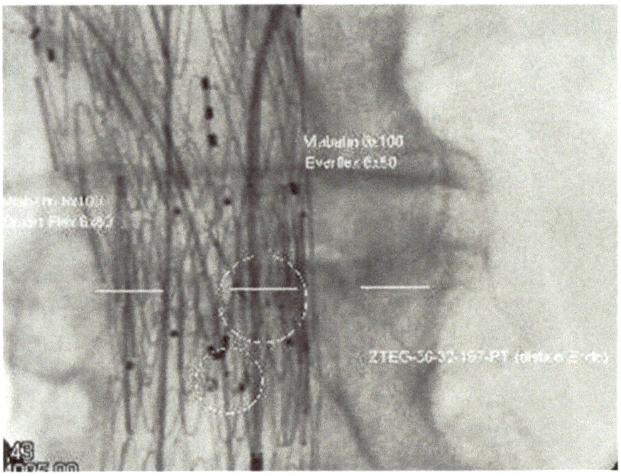

FIG. 13.8 Position of distal edge of the thoracic device.

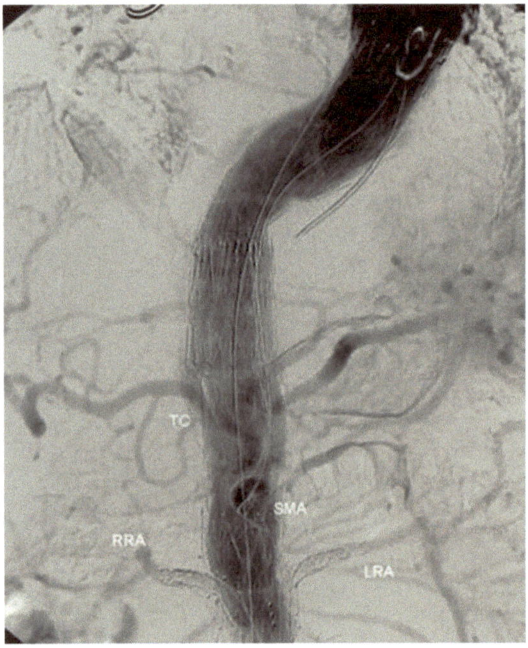

FIG. 13.9 Completion angiography after the treatment of the late type IA. *LRA*, Left renal artery; *RRA*, right renal artery; *SMA*, superior mesenteric artery; *TC*, celiac trunc.

In the presented case, we deployed a thoracic stent-graft between the primary descending aortic thoracic device and the fenestrated endograft. It is important to confirm the position of the distal edge of the thoracic device and its relation to the Viabahn grafts (Fig. 13.8).

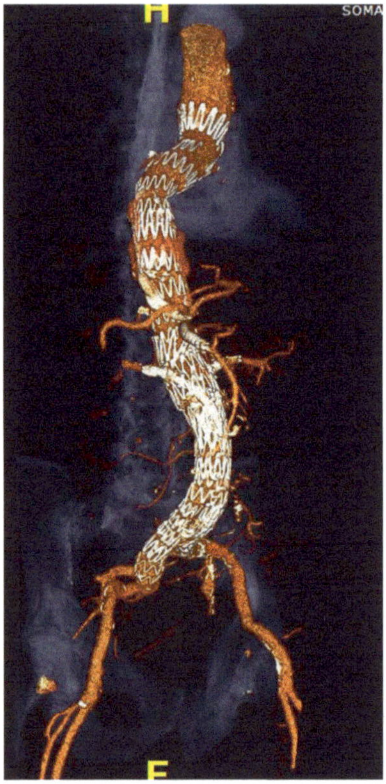

FIG. 13.10 Postoperative CTA reconstruction of the sandwich endovascular technique.

7. Placement of chimney grafts to the visceral arteries

Long Viabahn covered stents were deployed in the visceral vessels, each additionally lined with bare-metal self-expanding stents. We extended the devices above the proximal edge of the distal deployed thoracic device, creating a sandwich configuration.

Fig. 13.9 presents the final angiography of the treatment by the sandwich technique, without any evidence of gutter-related endoleaks. The postoperative CTA reconstruction confirmed patent chimney and periscope grafts, exclusion of the ruptured pathologic process, and no endoleaks (Fig. 13.10).

LIMITATIONS OF SANDWICH TECHNIQUE

Need for Upper Extremity Access

Deployment of renovisceral chimney grafts is associated with a few anatomic prerequisites.

The left subclavian artery must be patent if the plan is to deploy renal periscope grafts from the transfemoral access. In addition, the presence of soft plaque in the origin of the subclavian artery or descending aorta is associated with an increased risk of stroke. Monitoring of the ACT and additional administration of heparin to maintain an ACT of at least 250 seconds is mandatory.

The axillary artery must be large enough to accommodate at least two 8F sheaths. The 7 and 8 mm in diameter, self-expanding covered stents (Viabahn; Gore, Flagstaff, Arizona, USA) are compatible with an 8F sheath. This means that in the case of a calcified or a small-caliber axillary artery, introduction of two 8F sheaths is associated with a risk for peripheral occlusion and ischemia. When 10-mm Viabahn devices are required, an 11F sheath is necessary. Currently, the only available 10F sheaths compatible with a 10-mm Viabahn are the Cordis AVANTI Sheath, Boston Scientific Super Sheath, and the B. Braun Intradyn Tear-Away Sheath.

Absence of Dedicated Chimney Graft in Combination with Thoracic Device

Absence of a chimney graft is the major drawback of the technique. There are three main issues for a bridging chimney or periscope device when performing the sandwich technique: (1) the *length*, (2) the *radial force* of the device related to the thoracic stent-graft, and (3) the *comformability* of the thoracic endograft around the chimney graft. The Viabahn (Gore) covered stent addresses the issue of length in the sandwich technique. The device is available in several lengths between 5 and 25 cm, which allows extension into the thoracoabdominal aorta. Extrapolation of the results of in vitro study in the thoracic segment suggests that the combination of the Viabahn with the Gore thoracic device should be the first choice. This interaction seems to be ideal with respect to the radial force and the conformability of the thoracic device around the Viabahn.

LITERATURE REVIEW

Schwiertz et al.[1] reported in 2014 on 32 high-risk symptomatic patients with TAAAs treated by the sandwich technique. They found that a narrow aortic lumen is technically more demanding than a larger-diameter aorta. Placement of up to four chimneys into a calcified and narrow aorta should be avoided. Theoretically, this can cause aortic thrombosis as well as compromised perfusion of the chimney grafts. The authors recommend long-term antiplatelet therapy because, in contrast to a custom-made branched graft, reaccess of the Viabahn grafts after occlusion or in the presence of a high-grade stenosis can be very challenging or impossible.

Bisdas et al.[2] reported in 2013 a 68-year-old female patient with contained rupture of a 9-cm type III TAAA. An open repair was contraindicated on the basis of the patient's comorbid conditions, which included dialysis-dependent renal insufficiency, chronic obstructive pulmonary disease, coronary artery disease, and previous abdominal aortic repair. Because of hemodynamic instability, the patient underwent a totally endovascular repair with off-the-shelf devices using the sandwich technique. The patient's 12-month course was complicated by a gutter-related endoleak. An intraoperative gutter-associated endoleak resolved after 2 months. The 1-year CTA follow-up showed resolution of the endoleak between the outer and inner stent-graft layers. This staged evolution of the gutter-related endoleak until its complete disappearance, the first such presentation in the literature, confirmed the safety of the sandwich technique. The aneurysm was smaller in size and the visceral vessels were patent at the last follow-up visit.

REFERENCES

1. Schwiertz E, Kolvenbach RR, Yoshida R, et al. Experience with the sandwich technique in endovascular thoracoabdominal aortic aneurysm repair. *J Vasc Surg*. 2014;59:1562–1569.
2. Bisdas T, Donas KP, Bosiers M, et al. One-year follow-up after total endovascular repair of a contained-ruptured thoracoabdominal aortic aneurysm with the sandwich technique. *J Vasc Surg*. 2013;58(2):482–485.

CHAPTER 14

Thoracic Endovascular Aortic Repair

GIOVANNI FEDERICO TORSELLO

The treatment of thoracic aortic aneurysms depends on the location of the involved segment. Aneurysms of the ascending aorta and the arch are usually still treated by open repair, although endovascular solutions for these pathologies have been introduced in recent years. Ranging from hybrid procedures to parallel grafts and branched devices, treatment of the more proximal aortic segments will continue to evolve.

On the other hand, thoracic endovascular aortic repair (TEVAR) of aneurysms of the descending thoracic aorta (DTA) has become commonplace over the last several years. Compared with open repair, perioperative and short-term morbidity and mortality are lower with TEVAR.[1] Numerous reports on TEVAR results indicate that elderly patients and those with a high-risk profile especially benefit from this treatment, analogous to endovascular abdominal aneurysm repair (EVAR).

INDICATIONS

Corresponding with the treatment rationale for EVAR, the main goal of TEVAR is the exclusion of the aneurysm to prevent aneurysm rupture. Aneurysms with a diameter of 6 cm or more are considered to have a rupture risk of 10% to 15% and thus should be treated. Additional indications for DTA aneurysm repair include symptomatic and rapidly growing aneurysms as well as aneurysms with a saccular configuration.

PROCEDURE

Case Presentation

A 77-year-old patient presented with a 78-mm aneurysm of the DTA, increasing more than 10 mm in diameter in 1 year (Fig. 14.1). The patient had an open repair of an infrarenal abdominal aneurysm with a tube graft in 1998. A common iliac artery aneurysm on the right side had been treated by resection and interposition of a polyester prosthesis in 2005. In 2012 the patient underwent coronary artery bypass graft implantation for three-vessel coronary artery disease. Other relevant comorbidities were congestive heart failure, arterial hypertension, and a history of prostate cancer.

Preoperative Assessment

As with all patients for whom endovascular treatment is planned, this patient underwent a cardiology workup and duplex ultrasound evaluation of the carotid and peripheral arteries. Thin-sliced, arterial phased computed tomography angiography (CTA) is mandatory for preoperative planning of TEVAR procedures. This patient had an occlusion of the left internal carotid and the right vertebral artery. CTA of the intracranial arteries revealed that most of the brain parenchyma was perfused by the left vertebral artery (Fig. 14.2).

At our institution, St. Franziskus Hospital Münster, Germany, most surgeons use the Aquarius iNtuition software (TeraRecon, Foster City, California, USA) for preoperative planning. Other products (e.g., OsiriX; Pixmeo, Geneva) are equivalent, as long as they feature a centerline of flow function and multiplanar image reconstructions. The proximal landing zone, defined by the orifice of the left subclavian artery, was 46 mm long and kinked. The distal landing zone, defined by the orifice of the celiac trunk, was 42 mm long. The aortic segment between these sealing zones was tortuous, with several kinks.

Proximal neck diameter and angulation may be associated with inferior outcomes or may even prevent the deployment and fixation of the endograft. Depending on the choice of endograft, the instructions for use demand different maximum neck diameters and degrees of angulation. It is also important to assess access-vessel morphology, including minimal diameter, calcification, and tortuosity. At our institution, we always assess the level of the femoral bifurcations related to the femur heads. Based on this information, the adequate endograft is chosen, and the need for adjunctive procedures is assessed, such as subclavian-carotid transposition/bypass, chimney graft for left subclavian artery, iliofemoral conduits, or the paving-and-cracking technique.

Endograft Planning

Based on preoperative CTA, the surgeon creates a plan that often includes a sketch of the whole aorta, measuring proximal and distal neck lengths, assessing relevant aortic branches, and measuring the relevant diameters of the aorta and access vessels. If a large amount of thrombus is present, its localization is indicated in the drawing. Based on aortic morphology, the surgeon chooses the preferred endograft. Sizing of the endograft depends on the individual device. In this patient, we planned to implant a Zenith Alpha Thoracic Stent Graft (Cook Medical, Bloomington, Indiana, USA). We usually oversize this endograft by 20% because inadequate oversizing and undersizing carry the risk of type Ia endoleaks. The Zenith Alpha graft was chosen for this patient because of the aortic tortuosity. In our experience the major advantage of the Zenith Alpha is its flexibility and low profile, which greatly enhance trackability.[2]

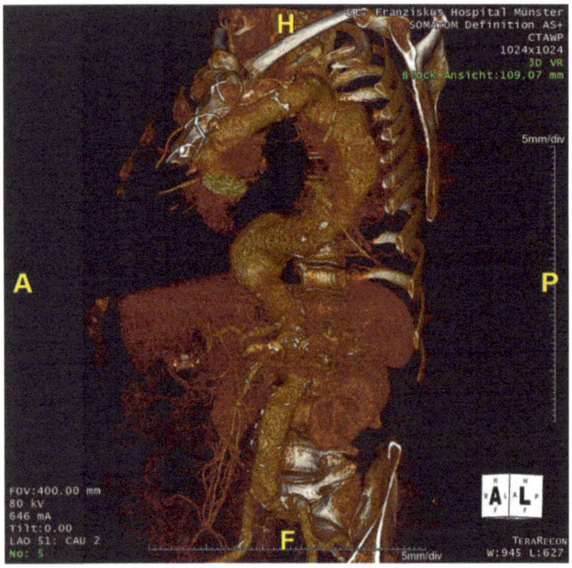

FIG. 14.1 Three-dimensional (3D) reconstruction of computed tomography angiogram (CTA) showing patient with 78-mm aneurysm of a tortuous descending thoracic aorta.

Access vessels

Compared with open repair, TEVAR is a more widely applicable treatment option, especially in relation to patient overall health status. In most cases, applicability of TEVAR is not limited by patient comorbidities, but rather by anatomic suitability. Access-vessel morphology is the Achilles' heel of TEVAR, especially when larger-bore sheaths are needed for smaller access vessels, as often seen in women and Asians, compared with EVAR devices, which are smaller bore. This translates to a higher rate of access vessel–related complications and the need for a more invasive access in TEVAR. Creation of an iliac conduit, either open or endovascular, can be a solution for challenging access. These

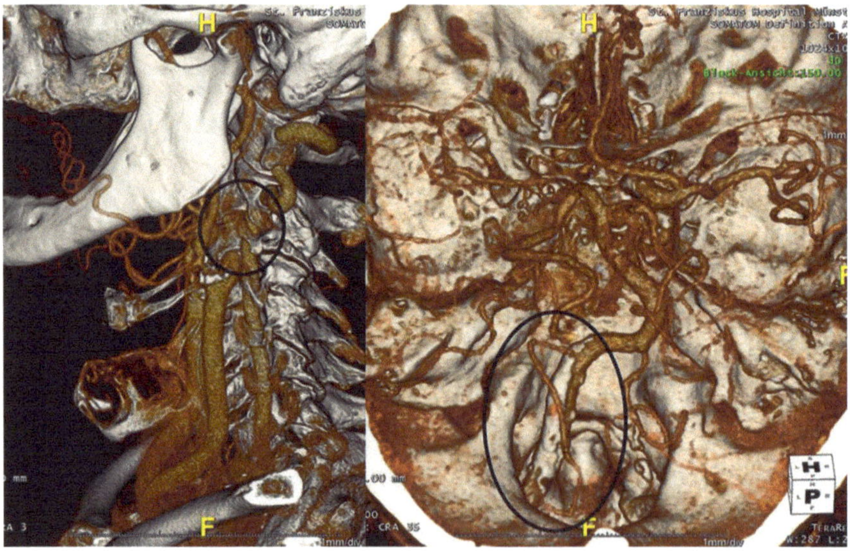

FIG. 14.2 3D reconstruction of CTA of the supra-aortic branches showing a proximal occlusion of the left internal carotid artery and a dominant left vertebral artery, feeding more than three quarters of the intracranial arteries.

and other techniques, however, have their own intrinsic morbidity and mortality.

At our institution, vessel access is usually completely percutaneous. After puncture of the common femoral arteries (CFAs), the preclose technique (Prostar XL, Abbott Vascular, Santa Clara, California, USA) was performed, with a 14-French (14F) sheath placed on the right side and an 8F sheath in the left CFA. Since the level of the femoral bifurcation in relation to the femoral heads is assessed beforehand, puncture of the CFA is usually safe, as in this patient.

In patients with small and diseased femoral vessels, we puncture the left brachial artery first. In the absence of contraindications, we prefer the left brachial, since we do not need to traverse the carotid arteries, reducing the incidence of embolic stroke.

After placement of a 5F Cook sheath, a 5F pigtail catheter is used to bring a standard Terumo wire (Radifocus Terumo, Japan) into the abdominal aorta. The pigtail catheter can be used to perform angiography of the iliofemoral axes and facilitate puncture of the CFAs (e.g., using the overlay function).

Deployment Preparation

During the procedure, intravenous heparin was administered to achieve an activated clotting time (ACT) corridor of 250 to 300 seconds. In this case, we used the pigtail catheter to mark the origin of the left subclavian artery (LSA), and a 5F Shepherd Hook catheter, advanced from the left femoral access, marked the orifice of the celiac trunk. From the right femoral access, we advanced a Lunderquist Extra-Stiff DC Wire Guide (Cook Medical) over a graded 5F pigtail catheter into the aortic root. In addition, we employed 2D/3D fusion imaging to facilitate the deployment of the endograft (see Chapter 20). The fusion imaging technique also assists in finding the appropriate projection to identify the maximally achievable proximal sealing zone and can aid in measuring the length of the aorta that needs to be sealed. The transbrachially placed pigtail catheter is then used to perform the initial CTA.

Stent-Graft Deployment

After validating the necessary graft length with a graded pigtail catheter and fusion imaging, the proximal component was deployed (Fig. 14.3). In this patient, as in almost all cases of DTA TEVAR, we used permissive hypotension of less than 80 mm Hg systolic blood pressure. We rarely use adenosine or rapid pacing to facilitate deployment.

Since the proximal hooks face distally, it is recommended to start the deployment a short distance distal to the intended landing zone. A positioning correction can be safe only when moving the endograft in a proximal direction.

Because of the dependence of cerebral perfusion on the left vertebral artery in this patient, coverage of the LSA was avoided. Even with less diseased cerebrovasculature, however, we usually avoid coverage of the LSA whenever possible. A number of studies have identified the higher risk of complications associated with LSA coverage, including arm claudication, subclavian steal syndrome, spinal cord ischemia, and stroke.[3] The transbrachially placed Terumo wire can be used for placement of a parallel graft in the event of intentional or inadvertent coverage of the LSA.

We also implanted a distal component, aiming for an overlap of at least three stents. We strongly advise against using two proximal components, since the distal component has barbs in the distal portion of the tube as a means of preventing migration.

Stent-graft conformability in tortuous aortic morphology

Together with the aforementioned access-vessel anatomy, the aortic morphology can be a major determinant of technical success. Recently introduced devices offer greatly improved conformability. A 2013 analysis of conformability of thoracic stent-grafts showed that the Valiant Captivia (Medtronic, Santa Clara, California, USA) was especially conformable to tortuous

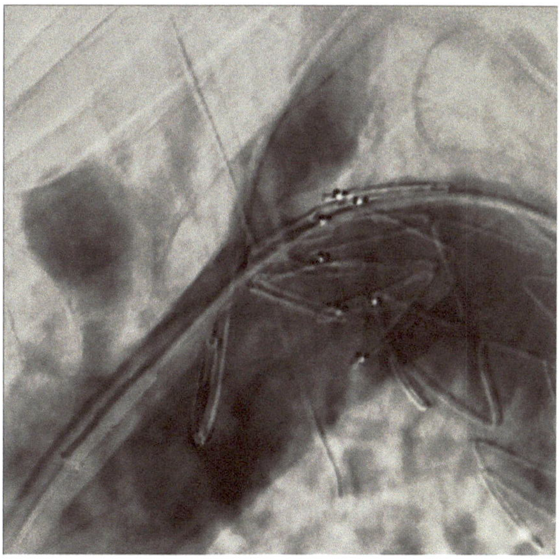

FIG. 14.3 Deployment of the proximal stent-graft component with a 5F pigtail catheter in the left subclavian artery to mark the proximal neck.

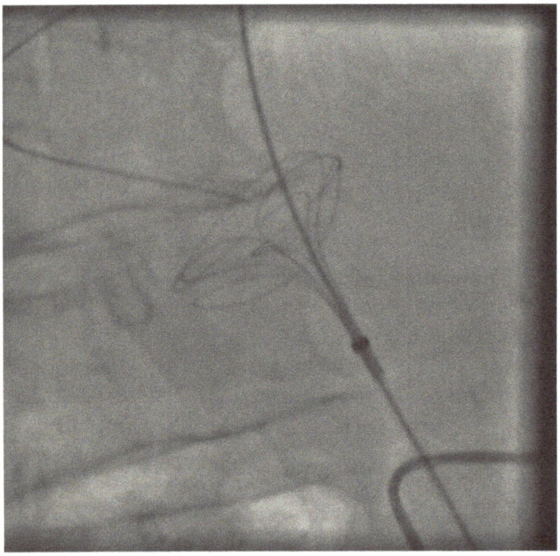

FIG. 14.4 Catching the pull-through wire with an Indy Snare Catheter.

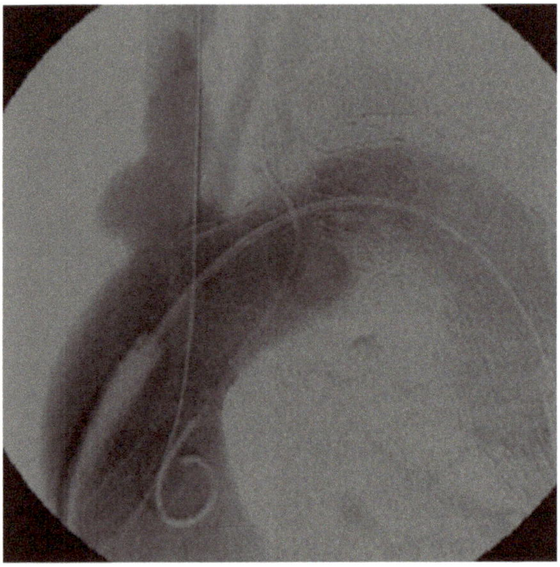

FIG. 14.5 Münster maneuver. To enhance stability, an extrastiff wire is advanced until a loop is created in the ascending aorta.

DTAs.[4] Recently, devices such as the Zenith Alpha and the Gore C-TAG were introduced, providing additional options to conform better to tortuous anatomies.[2,5]

In the present case, for example, the distal component could not be advanced into the proximal component because of the severe tortuosity. In a first step, we attempted to facilitate passage of the distal component by using a Reliant balloon (Medtronic) from the left femoral access. Molding the distal portion of the proximal component sometimes solves this problem. In this case, we had to advance the standard Terumo wire into the abdominal aorta and catch it with an Indy Snare Catheter (Cook Medical), utilizing it as a pull-through wire (Fig. 14.4). This through-and-through approach enabled us to deploy the distal component in the desired position, directly above the celiac trunk.

When necessary, we perform what we advocated as the "Münster maneuver," creating a loop in the ascending arch, which enhances stability especially for proximal deployment (Fig. 14.5). Another approach is the double-wire technique, with the placement of two extrastiff wires with or without additional stiff sheaths (e.g., 90-cm Destination Sheaths, Terumo). This can facilitate straightening of angled segments of the aortic segments close to the pathology.

In the presented case, a pull-through wire was sufficient to deploy the distal stent-graft component. A Reliant balloon was then used for stent-graft molding. After deployment of the graft, a completion angiogram was performed to ensure adequate placement of the graft and rule out endoleaks. The infrarenal aneurysm was then excluded in a standard manner (see Chapter 1). The arteriotomies were closed with the preclose sutures, and the brachial puncture site was manually compressed until bleeding control was achieved.

POSTOPERATIVE CARE

To prevent ischemic spinal cord injury, the patient's mean arterial blood pressure was maintained between 80 and 100 mm Hg for 48 hours postoperatively. Since we abandoned preventive drainage in 2013, we use cerebrospinal fluid drainage (CSFD) only in selected cases.

REFERENCES

1. Biancari F, Mariscalco G, Mariani S, et al. Endovascular treatment of degenerative aneurysms involving only the descending thoracic aorta: systematic review and meta-analysis. *J Endovasc Ther*. 2016;23(2):387–392.
2. Torsello GF, Austermann Martin, Van Aken Huko K, Torsello Giovanni B, Panuccio Giuseppe. Initial clinical experience with the Zenith Alpha stent-graft. *J Endovasc Ther*. 2015;22(2):153–159.

3. Hajibandeh S, Hajibandeh Shahab, Antoniou Stavros A, Torella Francesco, Antoniou George A. Meta-analysis of left subclavian artery coverage with and without revascularization in thoracic endovascular aortic repair. *J Endovasc Ther*. 2016;23(4):634–641.
4. Canaud L, Cathala Philipe, Joyeux Frédéric, Brancherau Pascal, Marty-Ané Charles, Alic Pierre. Improvement in conformability of the latest generation of thoracic stent grafts. *J Vasc Surg*. 2013;57(4):1084–1089.
5. Böckler D, Jan Brunkwall PR, Taylor N, Mangialardi J, Hüsing, Larzon Thomas. Thoracic endovascular aortic repair of aortic arch pathologies with the conformable thoracic aortic graft: early and 2 year results from a European mulicentre registry. *Eur J Vasc Endovasc Surg*. 2016;51:791–800.

CHAPTER 15

Branched Stent-Grafts in the Aortic Arch

KONSTANTINOS P. DONAS • MARTIN AUSTERMANN

The aortic arch is one of the most anatomically complex segments of the thoracoabdominal aorta because of the plurality of supra-aortic branch configurations and highly variable curvature. Endovascular treatment of aortic arch aneurysms using branched stent-grafts was reported initially by Inoue et al.[1] in 1999. Their device consisted of a unibody graft with up to three limbs that were snared and pulled into each of the aortic trunk vessels.

In 2003, Chuter et al.[2] described a modular branched stent-graft implanted proximally into the ascending aorta and distally into the innominate artery (IA) and descending thoracic aorta. However, this method has fallen out of favor due to various issues, including delivery of the device through the IA, size constraints, and relatively high stroke and mortality risk, approaching 30%. These factors, along with the success achieved in the thoracoabdominal aorta with branched stent-graft repair of thoraco-abdominal aneurysms, led to a refined design and revised thinking about the method of device introduction, resulting in a novel multibranched stent-graft intended for transfemoral insertion.

The branched stent-graft is custom-made (Cook Medical, Brisbane, Australia) and is available in diameters between 34 and 46 mm, with a covered length of 250 mm. The device is loaded into a Flexor sheath with a diameter of 20 to 24 French (F). Fig. 15.1 presents the curved delivery system.

The introducer has an inner nitinol cannula and is precurved. A notch in the dilator tip is aligned with the outer curve of the introducer and graft. The advantage of this novel introducer is that it automatically orients itself properly during placement into the arch without any rotational manipulation.

The graft is constructed with two side-branches (Fig. 15.2). Theoretically, a third branch could be added for the left subclavian artery (LSA). Usually, the branch for the left common carotid artery (LCCA) is an 8-mm side branch situated distally within the body of the graft at the 11:30 clock position, and the branch for the IA is a 12-mm branch situated proximal at the 12:30 position.

The first case with this device was performed in 2009 and involved a branched graft with external, funnel-shaped branches to facilitate their cannulation. In addition, the proximal stent was modified to incorporate the Cook Medical Pro-Form technology, so that proximal wall apposition was ensured. Gold markers indicated the location of side branches and the aspect of the graft to be aligned to the greater curve of the arch. Two sets of gold markers are placed at the branch entries: quadruple linear markers at the proximal edge of the innominate branch and the distal edge of the carotid branch entries, and double markers at the distal edge of the innominate branch and the proximal edge of the carotid branch entries. The stent-graft tapers at the site of the side-branch openings to provide more space to accommodate the branches.

Stent-grafts, such as Fluency (Bard Peripheral Vascular, Tempe, Arizona, USA) or Viabahn (W.L. Gore & Associates, Flagstaff, Arizona, USA), are used to bridge from the LCC side-branch to the LCCA. These bridging grafts require optional support with self-expanding stents. Because of the larger diameter of the IA, custom-made bridging limbs (Cook Medical) are used to bridge from the IA to its side branch (Fig. 15.3). These bridging

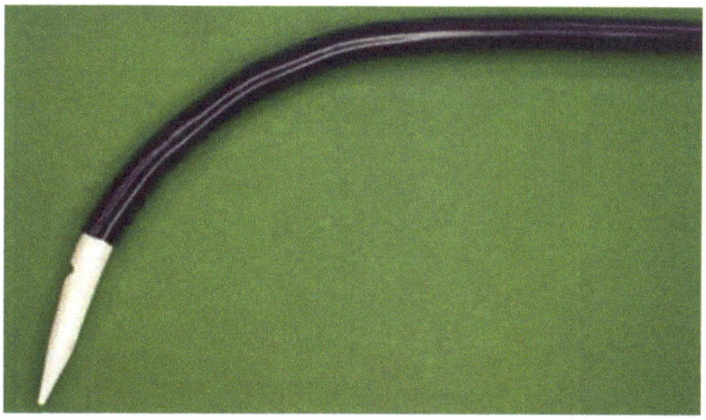

FIG. 15.1 The curved delivery system of the Flexor sheath.

limbs use 'low-profile" fabric and nitinol stents to ensure that the grafts can be loaded into a 14F flexor sheath.

INDICATIONS

- Elective asymptomatic aortic arch aneurysms

PROCEDURE

Case Presentation

A 77-year-old man presented with a 7.7-cm aneurysm of the aortic arch. The patient had severe chronic obstructive lung disease, arterial hypertension, and coronary artery disease. Further, he chose not to have open surgical repair. Fig. 15.4 shows the preoperative imaging and sizing.

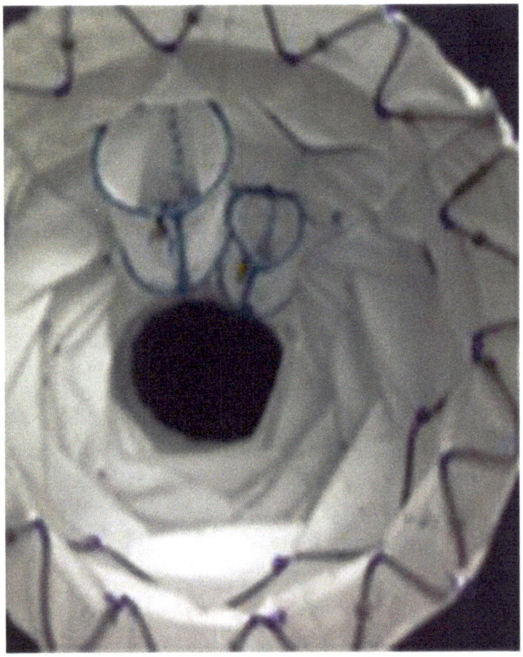

FIG. 15.2 The aortic arch graft with the two inner side branches.

Performance of Left Carotid–Subclavian Bypass

The origin of the LSA remains patent at this step of the procedure. The logic behind leaving the LSA patent is that the LCCA can often be closed to the IA, making cannulation of the inner branches of the arch device demanding or impossible. Having the orifice of the LSA patent simplifies cannulation via the LSA. In this particular case, the LCCA will be occluded with a vascular plug.

Insertion and Deployment of Branched Stent-Graft

The second step involves insertion of the branched stent-graft through femoral access. A double-curved, stiff Lunderquist guidewire is placed into the ascending aorta. The marker of the proximal and distal internal branches must lie proximal to the IA and LCCA ostia. Next, under rapid cardiac pacing, the sheath is withdrawn to expose the graft completely. The first three release rings are pulled on the control handle to sequentially deploy the device. The branches for the IA and LCCA are then cannulated through the right- and the left-sided sheath, respectively; while the fourth release ring remains in place to retain the distal attachment and stabilize the graft. Bridging of the IA is accomplished with a custom-made limb, which can be introduced through the right axillary artery or through a conduit sewn onto it (Fig. 15.5).

Insertion of Stents

A covered stent is used for bridging of the LCCA or LSA, and this may be further supported with a bare-metal self-expanding stent. In this case, we used a self-expanding covered stent (Fluency). At the end of the procedure and after successful cannulation of the LCCA, a 22-mm Amplatzer Plug (St. Jude) was placed in the LSA. Fig. 15.6 presents the placement of the covered stent in the LCCA and the occlusion of the LSA orifice by the vascular plug.

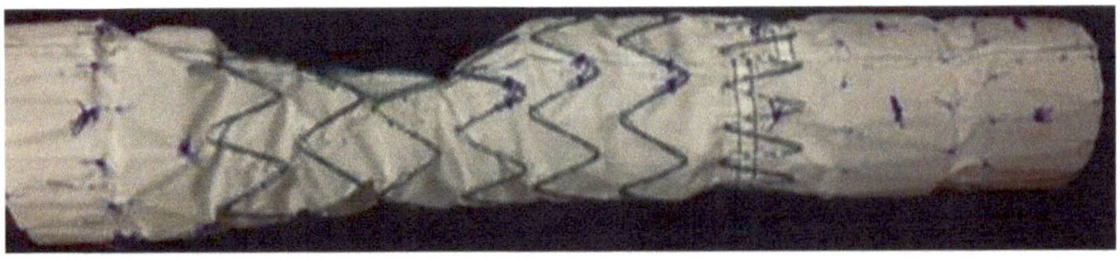

FIG. 15.3 Presentation of the aortic arch branched device based on the Zenith (Cook Medical) platform.

Completion and Follow-up Imaging

The final angiogram showed exclusion of the aneurysm and a patent carotid-subclavian bypass (Fig. 15.7). In addition, the 12-month postoperative computed tomography (CT) follow-up showed no evidence of endoleak and confirmed a patent carotid-subclavian bypass (Fig. 15.8).

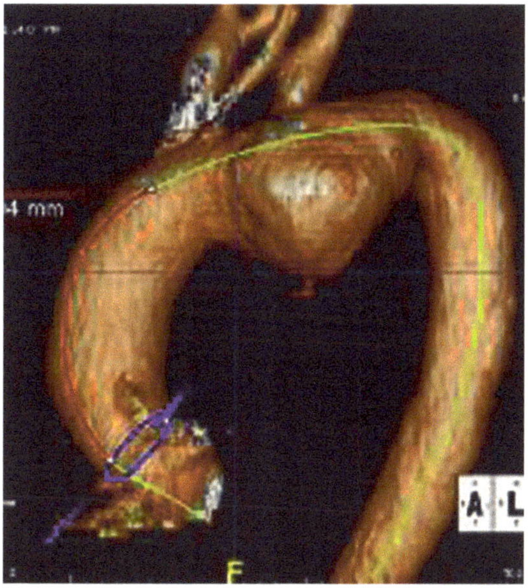

FIG. 15.4 Preoperative imaging of the aortic arch.

LIMITATIONS OF BRANCHED STENT-GRAFT

The risk of stroke in these patients remains high. Complex arch anatomy may necessitate extensive manipulation within the arch during positioning of the stent-graft or during cannulation of branches. Strokes may be embolic or result from inadequate cerebral perfusion. Therefore, excessive arch calcification or thrombus formation ("shaggy" aorta) should be considered high-risk conditions for neurologic events.

In addition, endografts placed in the ascending aorta and the aortic arch are subject to high-pulsatile forces that may affect their structural integrity. In the absence of adequate long-term durability data, the aortic arch branched stent-grafts should currently be limited to patients with ascending aortic diameter less than 38 mm, because the largest available proximal graft diameter is 46 mm. However, many of the patients presenting with arch disease have an ascending aortic diameter that exceeds 38 mm. Landing in a large, unhealthy ascending aorta may be associated with an increased rate of complications in the long term.

Lastly, the branched aortic arch stent-grafts are large, requiring a 24F (inner diameter) sheath for a 46-mm graft. These larger-profile systems have been associated with increased access site complications and an increase in the need for vascular cutdowns and conduits.[3]

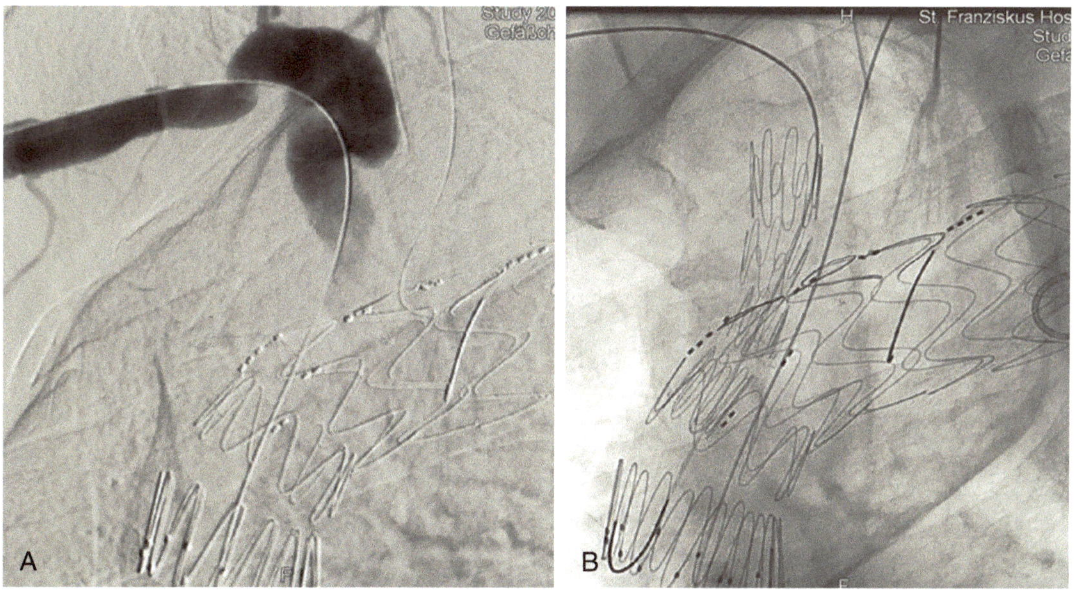

FIG. 15.5 **A, B,** Cannulation of the innominate artery from the right axillary artery and deployment of the custom-made limb device in the first branch.

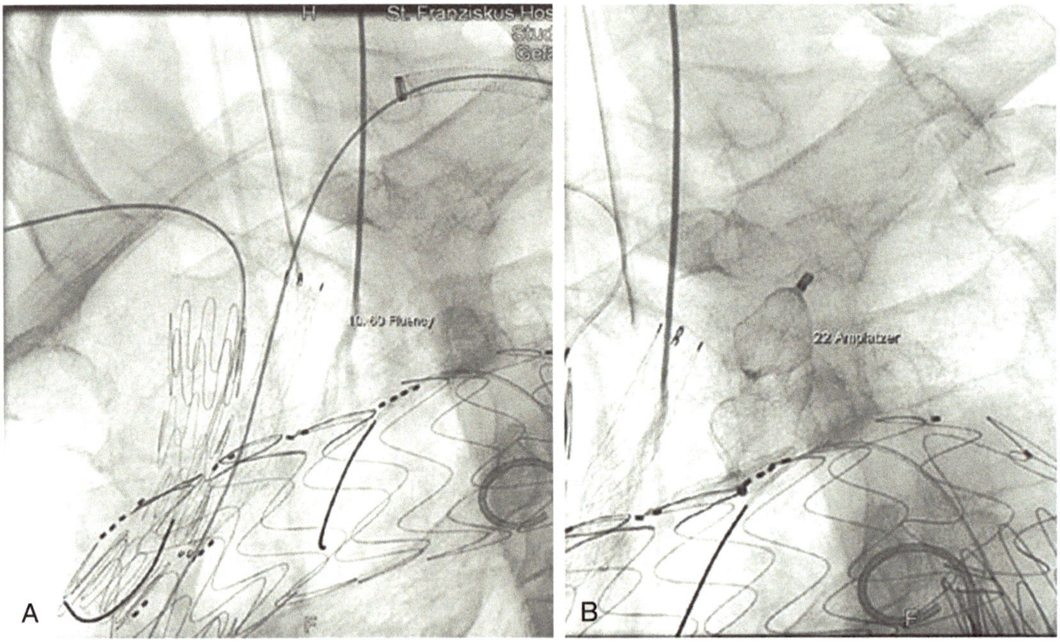

FIG. 15.6 **A,** Deployment of the self-expanding covered stent (Fluency) in the left common carotid artery. **B,** Occlusion of the left subclavian artery at the origin by a 22-mm Amplatzer Plug (St. Jude).

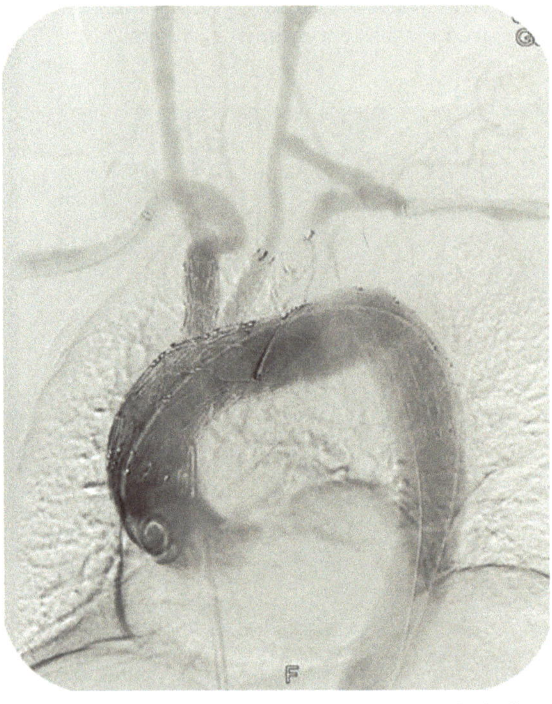

FIG. 15.7 Final angiogram shows the patent arch device and supra-aortic branches, without evidence of an endoleak.

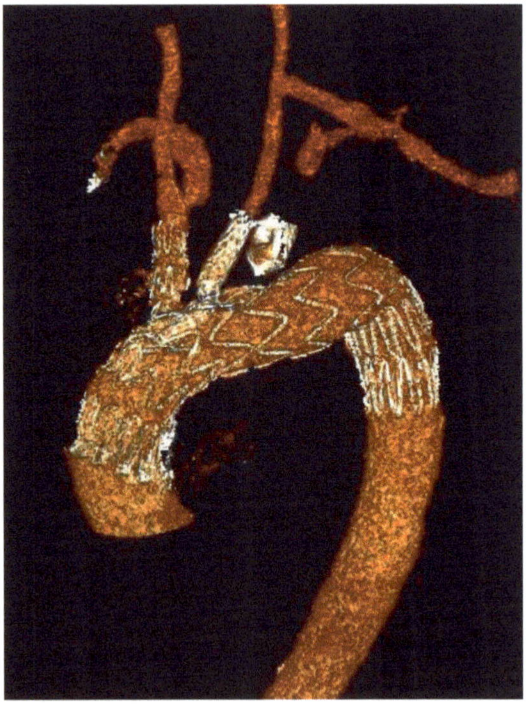

FIG. 15.8 The 12-month postoperative CT reconstruction with the aortic arch device.

LITERATURE REVIEW

In 2012, Lioupis et al.[4] first reported the technical feasibility of the branched stent-graft for treatment of aortic arch aneurysms. In this series of six patients, four had uneventful placement of the prostheses, with successful exclusion of their aneurysms. In one patient a type I endoleak developed, which was managed successfully with coiling and gluing of the aneurysm sac. In one patient, cannulation of the innominate branch was unsuccessful, and an extra-anatomic bypass was necessary to perfuse the right carotid and vertebral arteries; in this patient a stroke developed. Another patient had a right cerebellar infarct.

In 2014, Haulon et al.[5] reported a global registry of 38 patients treated with this arch branch graft; technical success was achieved in 32 patients (84.2%). Technical failures included three deaths within 24 hours of the procedure, one type Ia endoleak, one failure to cannulate the IA branch, and one conversion to a chimney technique. Five patients (13.2%) died within 30 days of the procedure, and there were six cerebrovascular complications in follow-up, including four transient ischemic attacks, one completed stroke, and one subarachnoid hemorrhage. Mortality was 30% in the first 10 patients and 7.1% in the subsequent 28 patients. Poor outcome was associated with large aortic diameter. Patients with ascending aortic diameter greater than 38 mm had a greater risk of stroke and death than those with smaller ascending aortas ($P = 0.026$). This initial study demonstrated the feasibility of total endovascular arch repair. The authors conclude that with proper operator training and careful patient selection, aortic arch repair can be extended to this difficult patient group who have been excluded from surgical or other endovascular treatment.

REFERENCES

1. Inoue K, Hosokawa H, Iwase T, et al. Aortic arch reconstruction by transluminally placed endovascular branched stent graft. *Circulation*. 1999;100(19 suppl):II316e21.
2. Chuter TA, Schneider DB, Reilly LM, Lobo EP, Messina LM. Modular branched stent graft for endovascular repair of aortic arch aneurysm and dissection. *J Vasc Surg*. 2003; 38(4):859e63.
3. Maurel B, Mastracci TM, Spear r, et al. Branched and fenestrated options to treat aortic arch aneurysms. *J Cardiovasc Surg*. 2016;57:686–697.
4. Lioupis C, Corriveau MM, MacKenzie KS, Obrand DI, Steinmetz OK, Abraham CZ. Treatment of aortic arch aneurysms with a modular transfemoral multibranched stent graft: initial experience. *Eur J Vasc Endovasc Surg*. 2012;43:525–532.
5. Haulon S, Greenberg RK, Spear R, et al. Global experience with an inner branched arch endograft. *J Thorac Cardiovasc Surg*. 2014;148:1709–1716.

Chimney Thoracic Endovascular Technique

MICHEL BOSIERS • KONSTANTINOS P. DONAS • MARIO LACHAT

Lesions in the aortic arch or descending aorta can be treated using open or endovascular methods. When the lesion is located close to or involves the supra-aortic branches, treatment becomes more difficult, and hybrid approaches may be necessary. In such cases, *debranching* must be performed to create an adequate landing zone for the thoracic endograft. The requirement for more than one procedure in hybrid cases makes them less attractive than total endovascular repair with, for example, custom-made branched or fenestrated endografts. The obligatory delay between stages of a hybrid treatment comes with a high cost. With these limitations in mind, the chimney technique was developed as a total, one-stage endovascular solution to treat urgent and acute pathologies with off-the-shelf devices. (See also Chapters 6 to 8.)

PROCEDURE

Case Presentation

A 77-year-old woman presented with a contained rupture of an aortic arch aneurysm. A total endovascular repair using the chimney technique was elected. Fig. 16.1 shows the ruptured aortic arch, as well as a lusoria artery (aberrant subclavian artery).

Exposure of left axillary/proximal brachial artery

The patient's arm was abducted to 90 degrees. The proximal brachial artery was exposed through a 3- to 4-cm longitudinal incision in the groove between biceps and triceps, distally to the attachment of the pectoralis major muscle. The axillary (or proximal brachial) artery was carefully exposed, taking care to avoid injury of the median nerve, and prepared for puncture along its ventral surface. This approach facilitates the use of 7-French (7F) or 8F sheaths. Alternatively, when a single chimney graft is required, a percutaneous approach to the brachial artery in the antecubital fossa can also be performed. We recommend this only with planned placement of bare-metal stents as chimney grafts, since they are compatible with sheaths less than 7F in size.

Puncture of left brachial artery and cannulation of subclavian artery

The axillary artery is punctured using Seldinger technique, and after insertion of a short 5F sheath, 5000 units of heparin is administered. The next step is the insertion of the soft Terumo wire in the aortic arch and the advance of a 5F pigtail catheter in the ascending aorta, followed by a 7F sheath (Fig. 16.2).

Percutaneous transfemoral access

As in standard thoracic endovascular aneurysm repair (TEVAR), stiff wires are advanced using the Prostar XL device (Abbott).

Deployment of the thoracic endograft

Thoracic endografts are used per the center's standard, including devices with stainless steel or nitinol endoskeletons. The thoracic device will cover the orifice of the left subclavian artery and part of the orifice of the next supra-aortic vessel. The sheath is placed in the ascending aorta proximal to the covered part of the thoracic device (Fig. 16.3). Note the position of the C-arm in 30-degree left anterior oblique (LAO) position and the magnification of the images.

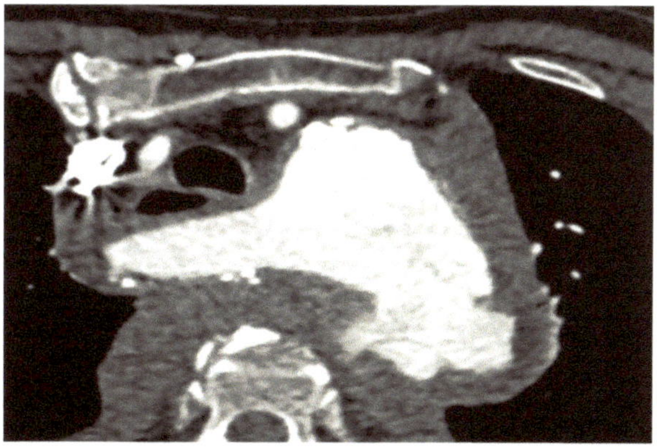

FIG. 16.1 Ruptured aortic arch aneurysm.

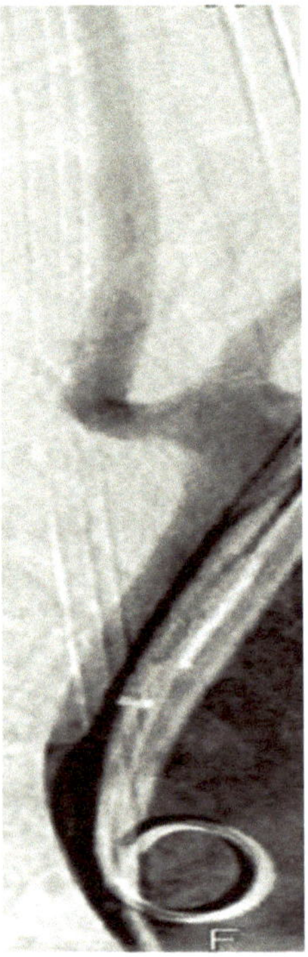

FIG. 16.2 Placement of the pigtail catheter in the ascending aorta via the 7F shuttle sheath using a telescope technique. The pigtail catheter is used for angiography. The sheath is placed in the ascending aorta for the subsequent advancement of the chimney graft.

After placement of the thoracic device, a stiff wire with an atraumatic tip such as the Rosen wire (Cook Medical) or Advantage wire (Terumo) is advanced over the brachial sheath. This provides a stable position for the deployment of the chimney graft. Fig. 16.4 shows deployment of an 8-mm-diameter, 59-mm-long Advanta/i-Cast V12 (Maquet) balloon-expandable covered stent in the left subclavian artery (LSA). The device will be placed parallel to and outside of the thoracic device.

The aneurysm exclusion based on the completion angiography (Fig. 16.5) was confirmed by computed tomography angiography (CTA) postoperatively (Figs. 16.6 and 16.7).

Modification of chimney technique in aortic arch by placement of self-expanding covered stents in left subclavian artery as periscopes

Professor Mario Lachat and the Zurich group suggest the placement of periscope grafts (reversed chimney grafts) in the LSA from the transfemoral access. Because of the need for long devices, the Viabahn covered

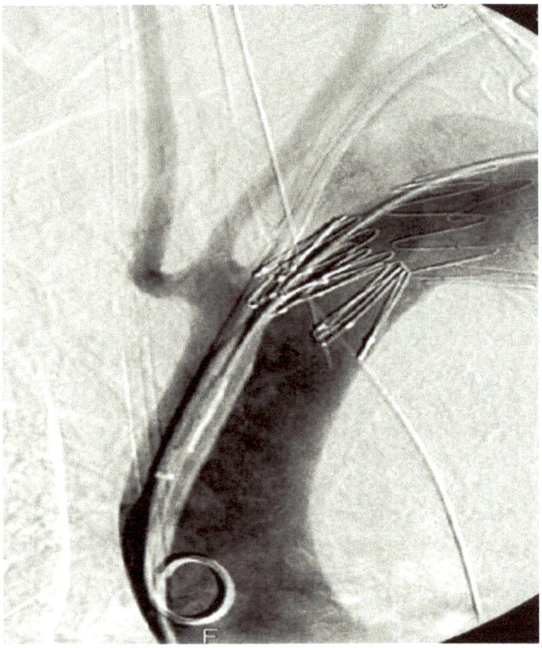

FIG. 16.3 Deployment of the thoracic endograft covering the left subclavian artery and, in this case, lusoria artery. The transbrachial sheath remains in the ascending aorta to advance the chimney graft. Note that this patient has a bicarotid trunk.

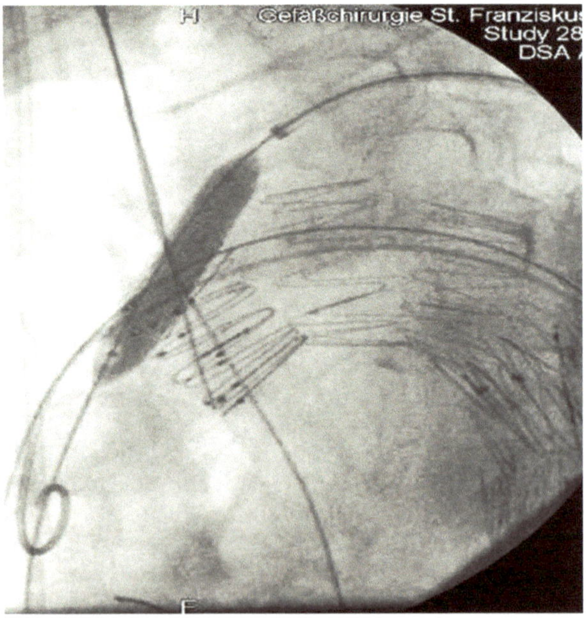

FIG. 16.4 Successful placement of the chimney balloon-expandable covered stent in the left subclavian artery after deployment of the thoracic endograft.

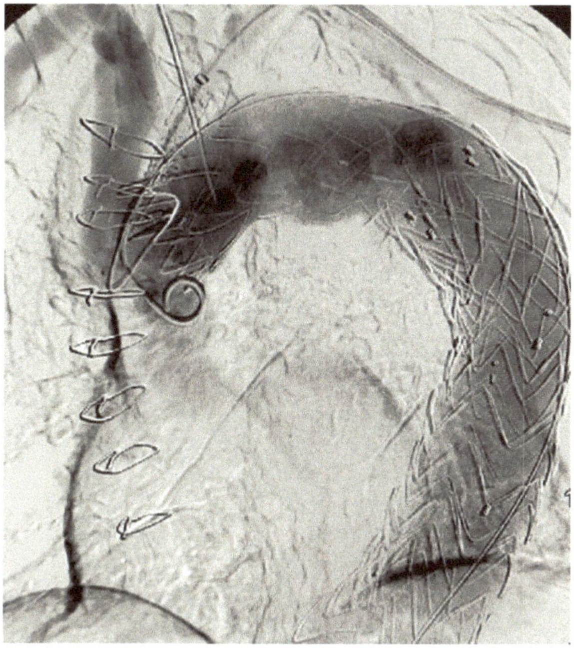

FIG. 16.5 Completion angiogram without evidence of type Ia endoleak and with successful exclusion of the aneurysm.

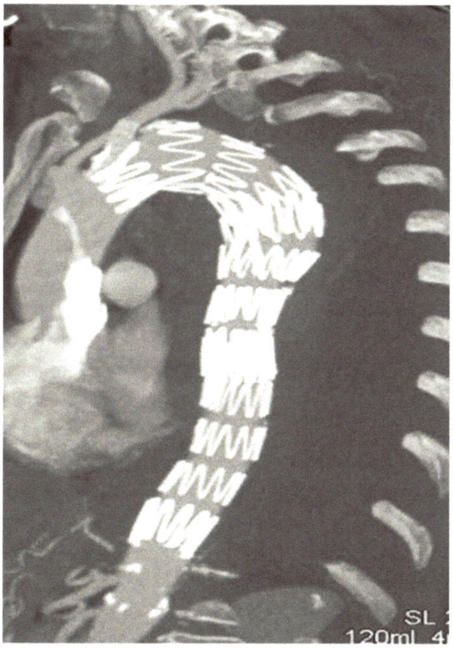

FIG. 16.6 Reconstruction of the postoperative computed tomography angiogram.

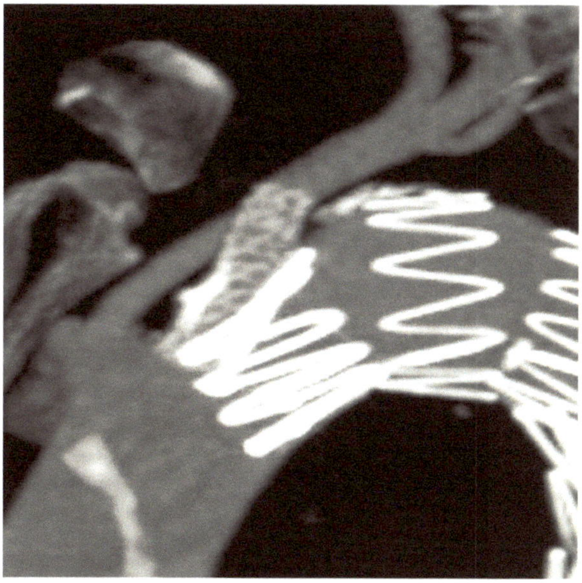

FIG. 16.7 Configuration of the balloon-expandable covered stent and the rigid stainless steel endoskeleton of the deployed thoracic device.

stent, available in lengths up to 250 mm, is used. This approach avoids placement of parallel grafts in the aortic arch, which is a segment with high pressure and in combination with a "bird beak" anatomy can be a significant risk for type Ia endoleak.

The suggested technique allows placement of only one device in the aortic arch, improving the conformability and minimizing the risk for chimney graft migration, gutter leaks, and type Ia endoleak. The chimney graft is positioned as a periscope device, originating in the descending thoracic aorta and terminating in the LSA.

Fig. 16.8 illustrates the planned technique for a pathologic process involving the aortic arch, with complete debranching of the supra-aortic vessels and periscope graft placement for the LSA.

The technique consists of the following:

- Ultrasound-guided microaccess puncture of the left axillary artery is performed. The arm position is in abduction with the hand behind the head.
- An 8F sheath with a 0.0014- or 0.0018-inch guidewire is introduced, which will be snared in the ascending or the descending aorta and exteriorized through the common femoral artery.
- A 9F sheath is advanced in the femoral artery. A through-and-through guidewire is used to exchange the thin guidewire for an Amplatz stiff guidewire (Fig. 16.9).

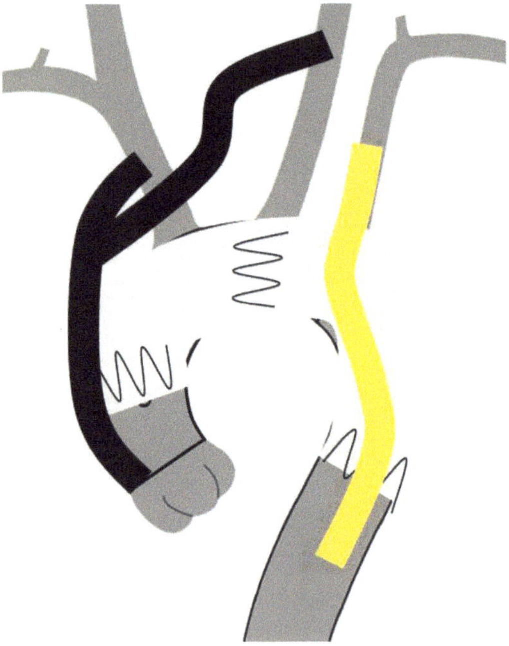

FIG. 16.8 Illustration of periscope technique, with *yellow* for the left subclavian artery. The patient also underwent complete debranching of the supra-aortic vessels.

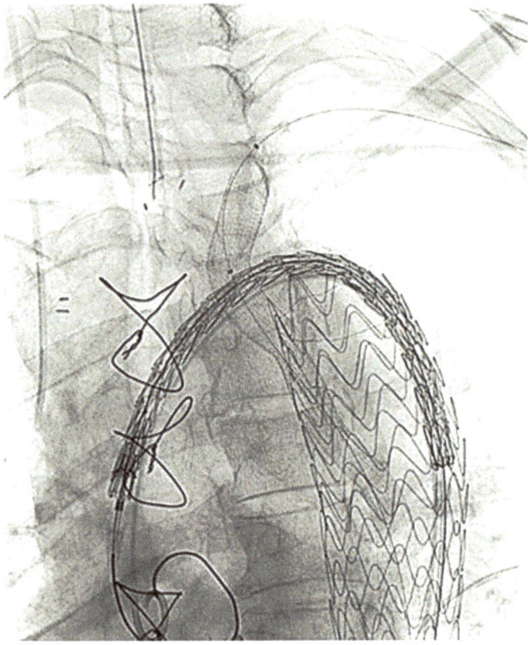

FIG. 16.10 Deployed thoracic device with the Viabahn in place.

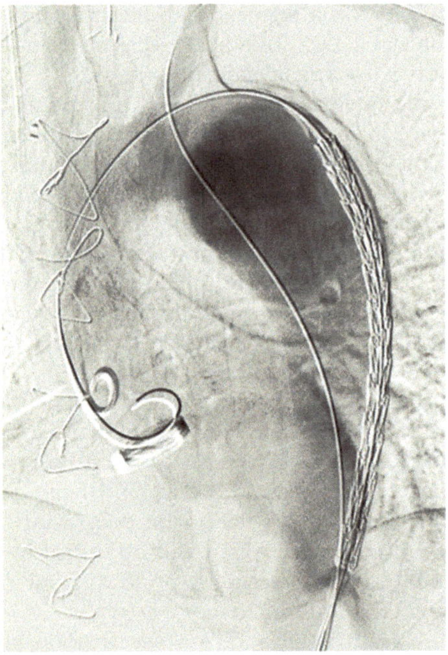

FIG. 16.9 Advancement of the thoracic device over the stiff wire and the previously placed (transfemoral) wire in the left subclavian artery.

- Generally, the 9F femoral sheath is exchanged for a 12F and 80-cm-long sheath (e.g., Cook Medical), and the Viabahn device (Gore) is parked in the proximal LSA.
- The aortic stent-graft is introduced and deployed from the contralateral femoral artery access (Fig. 16.10).

Lastly, the periscope is constructed by deploying the Viabahn device, reinforced with wall stents of appropriate length and diameter (Fig. 16.11).

LITERATURE REVIEW

Hogendoorn et al.[1] reported a meta-analysis of studies on the chimney technique in the treatment of aortic arch pathology. The interventions were elective in 72% and emergent in 28% of patients. Technical success was achieved in 98% of the treated patients. Type Ia endoleaks were reported in 6.4%. Stroke was reported in 5.3% of patients, of which 40% were fatal. Limitations of this meta-analysis include a lack of detailed information about the types of chimney grafts used in 13% of patients and no description of follow-up frequency in 45%.

Bosiers et al.[2] collected the current European experience with imaging follow-up for all patients and a detailed description of all used devices. The midterm

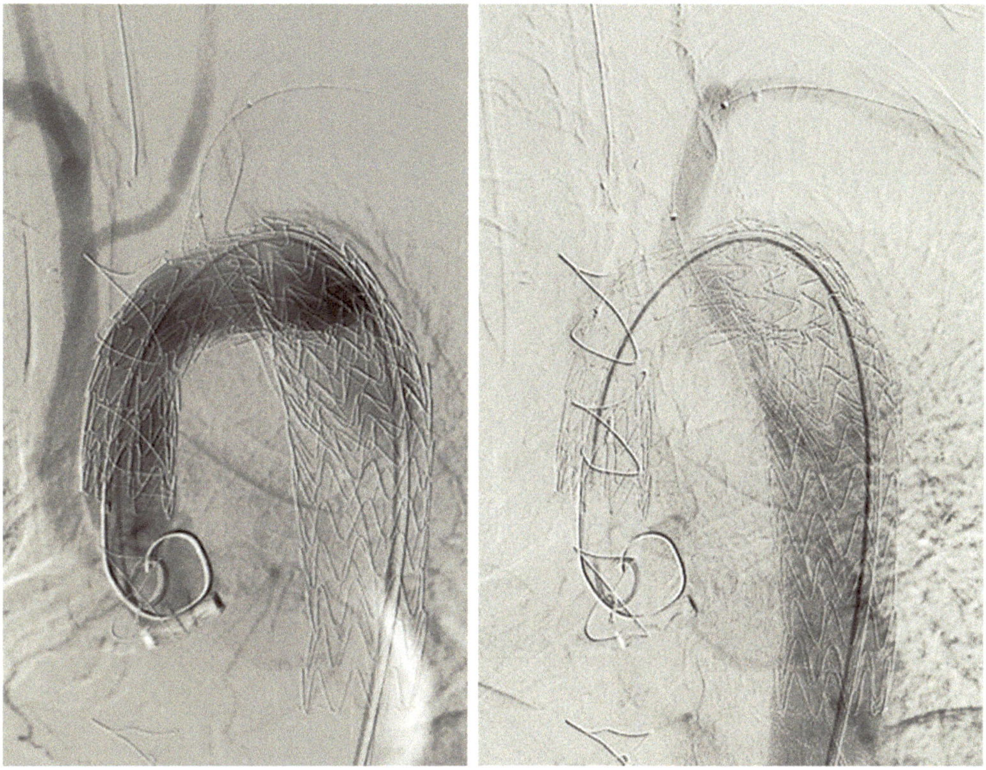

FIG. 16.11 Completion angiograms showing patent debranched supra-aortic vessels and left subclavian artery and periscope graft.

results confirmed a high rate of technical success and a low incidence of reinterventions, highlighting the utility of the chimney thoracic endovascular technique, especially for clinical indications that require urgent treatment. The increase of the neck length from 6.9 mm preoperatively to 26.5 mm postoperatively by placement of chimney grafts in the involved supra-aortic branches led to sufficient exclusion of the pathologies and only rare cases of persistent type Ia endoleak. Combination of the thoracic TAG (Gore) and Valiant (Medtronic) devices with self-expanding covered stents and balloon-expandable covered stents, respectively, shows better conformability, minimizing the area of the gutters and thus the risk of type Ia endoleaks.

Lessons learned from the current experience revealed that creation of a minimum 20-mm sealing-zone length is mandatory to reduce the risk for gutter-related type I endoleak. The underlying thought is that the longer the overlap, the faster the occlusion of the gutters, because of better adaptation of the endograft around the chimney stent-graft.

LIMITATIONS OF CHIMNEY TECHNIQUE

The major issues with the chimney thoracic endovascular technique include the incidence of gutter-related endoleaks and the risk for stroke because of the access from the upper extremity. Bosiers et al.[2] showed in the European chimney registry that 50% of the primary type Ia endoleaks resolved spontaneously within the first month postoperatively. Only 5.4% of all treated patients underwent secondary procedures for a persistent type I endoleak. Four of these five patients were symptomatic. Proximal extension or embolization was performed. The stroke rate was 4.2%, similar to previous reported stroke rates using hybrid approaches.

REFERENCES

1. Hogendoorn W, Schlösser FJ, Moll FL, et al. Thoracic endovascular aortic repair with the chimney graft technique. *J Vasc Surg*. 2013;58(2):502–511.
2. Bosiers MJ, Donas KP, Mangialardi N, et al. European Multicenter Registry for the performance of the chimney/snorkel technique in the treatment of aortic arch pathologic conditions. *Ann Thorac Surg*. 2016;101(6):2224–2230.

Bridging Devices in Complex Endovascular Aneurysm Repair

KONSTANTINOS P. DONAS • KENNETH OURIEL

Numerous bridging devices have been used in patients undergoing complex endovascular aneurysm repair (EVAR) with involvement of one or more target vessels. In this chapter we highlight the most common bridging devices and outline their strengths and limitations, as used in the Department of Vascular Surgery at St. Franziskus Hospital Münster, Germany.

STAINLESS STEEL BALLOON-EXPANDABLE COVERED STENTS

The Advanta/i-Cast V12 (Maquet) was designed based on the polytetrafluoroethylene (PTFE) film-covering technology. The 316L stainless steel struts are completely covered on their luminal and abluminal surfaces, protecting both the flow lumen and the wall from contact with the struts. In addition , the double coverage prevents disconnection of the stents struts from the PTFE material, preventing injury or dissection of the target vessels. The open-cell design facilitates safe advancement through sheaths, particularly in an angulated descending aorta, minimizing the risk of stent loss from the balloon. This complication was reported in the past, since the first-generation covered stents had a closed-cell design.

Fig. 17.1 shows the stainless steel balloon-expandable covered stent (BECS). The length of covered stents in fenestrated/branched (f/b-EVAR) and chimney (ch-EVAR) endovascular repair varies from 22 to 38 to 59 mm. The devices are compatible with a 7-French (7F) sheath and have diameters ranging between 5 and 8 mm.

Features

Key features include radial force and fluoroscopic visibility.

Radial force

The radial force of the bridging devices plays an important role. High radial force is essential to maintain long-term patency when bridging devices are used parallel to and outside of abdominal or thoracic devices. Computed tomography angiography (CTA) shows the ideal conformability of the Endurant device around the three balloon-expandable chimney grafts. The covered stents are completely expanded, achieving the intended nominal diameter without compression. Such observations make stainless steel BECSs the first choice in the chimney technique, particularly in combination with the Endurant abdominal stent-graft system.

Fluoroscopic visibility

Good fluoroscopic visibility is the next important feature which characterizing the Advanta BECS (Fig. 17.2A). The proximal and distal edge of the device can be

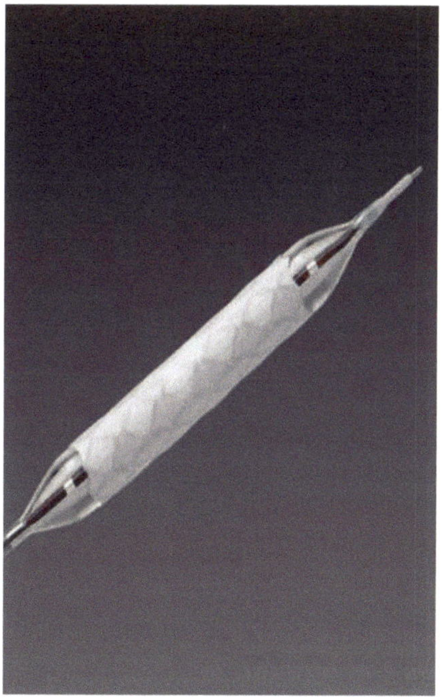

FIG. 17.1 Advanta/i-Cast balloon-expandable covered stent.

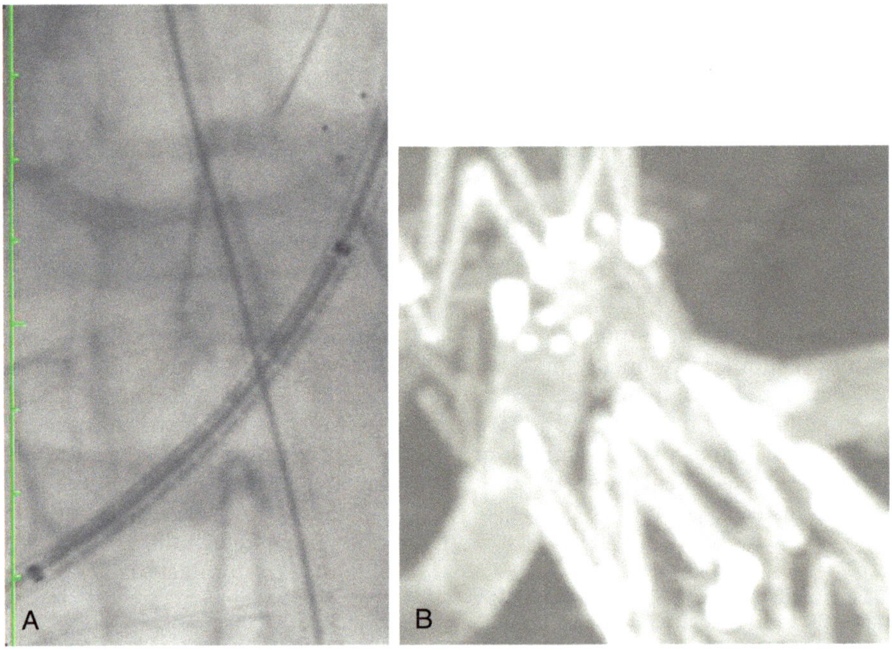

FIG. 17.2 **A,** Proximal and distal edges of the balloon-mounted covered stent. **B,** Ideal placement of the chimney graft in the middle of the suprarenal stent of the aortic endograft.

easily identified during the procedure, especially when the operation is performed in a hybrid angiosuite with advanced imaging equipment. Adequate imaging is imperative for precise positioning of the covered stent.

Adequate fluoroscopic visibility plays an important role when the Advanta covered stent is deployed in conjunction with the Endurant stent-graft in a parallel chimney configuration. The goal is to deploy the device in the middle of the suprarenal stent of the endograft (Fig. 17.2B). Fig. 17.3 shows the potential risk for interaction and cutting of the balloon from the pins of the suprarenal stent of the Endurant device.

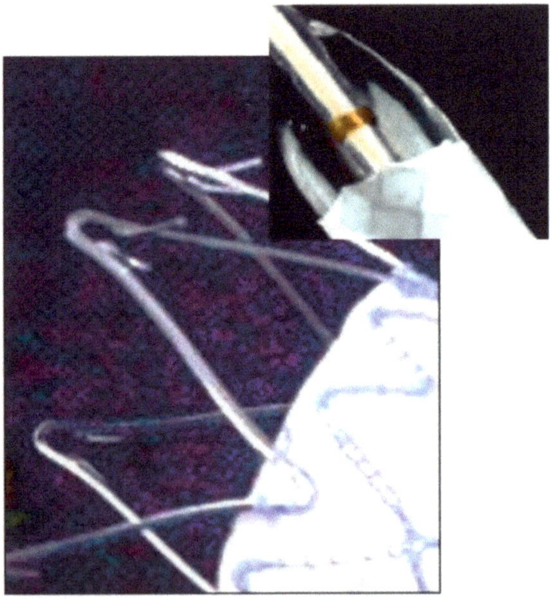

FIG. 17.3 Pins of suprarenal stent of Endurant device. The pins have the potential to cut the balloon of the chimney graft and provoke an uncontrolled interaction between the abdominal device and graft.

Limitations

The balloon-expandable devices are rigid. In angulated renal arteries, this rigidity requires lining with additional, self-expanding, flexible nitinol stents to improve the transition of the device. Fig. 17.4 illustrates the smooth transition of the BECS in angulated anatomy after lining with deployment of a nitinol bare-metal stent.

Literature Review

Chimney technique

Stainless steel BECSs were deployed in 49.2% (442) of 898 target aortic branch vessels in the worldwide collected experience on the use of chimney grafts

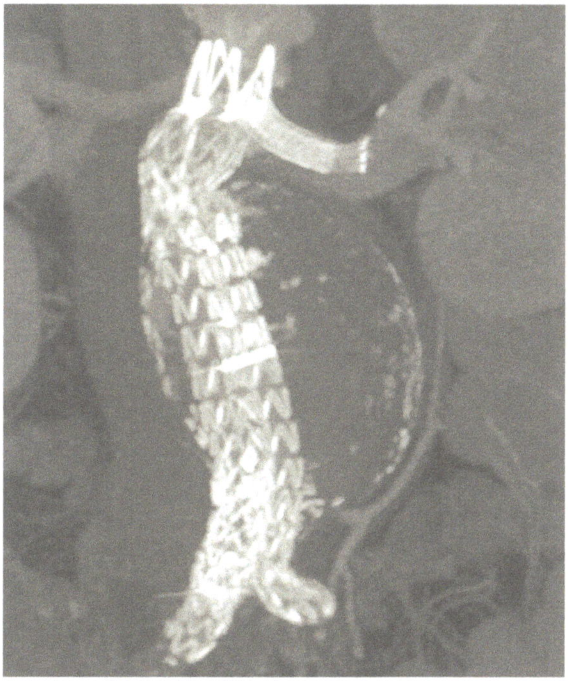

FIG. 17.4 Combined placement of balloon-expandable chimney covered stent proximally and a self-expanding nitinol bare-metal stent distally in the renal artery, achieving a smooth transition of the chimney graft in an angulated renal artery.

(PERICLES Registry).[1] In vitro testing recommended the combination of the Endurant device with the Advanta/i-Cast V12. The results of the PROTAGORAS Study confirmed the combination of Endurant and Advanta and are in agreement with the in vitro experience from the Barcelona group, for more than 120 patients. The freedom from new-onset type I endoleaks requiring reintervention was 98.4%.[2]

Fenestrated endovascular technique

Panuccio et al.[3] reported the Münster experience with stainless steel BECSs in fenestrated and branched endografting; 150 consecutive patients underwent f/b-EVAR, and 523 target vessels were treated, including 104 celiac, 140 superior mesenteric (SMA), 275 renal, and 4 other arteries. The technical success rate was 99% (520 of 523 target vessels). BECSs were most frequently used (95%). Lining with additional stents was used in 336 patients (65%).

After a median follow-up of 14 months, 13 (2%) bridging stent-grafts (BSGs) occluded and 19 (4%) required reintervention. Two SMA occlusions occurred, leading to death in both patients. The 3-year patency rate was 85%. The composite outcome of freedom from reintervention and occlusion of the bridging device was 80% at 3 years. Of note, the use of relining stents seemed not to prevent BSG-related complications.

Mastracci et al.[4] reported a freedom from reintervention and occlusion rate of 89% at 3 years. However, only the first event in each patient was recorded in this analysis, and multiple reinterventions related to BSGs were not separately reported. This may bias the results, considering that multiple secondary procedures in each patient can underestimate the rate of events. In contrast, a per-branch analysis on the basis of an intention-to-treat protocol was performed in the Münster study. In this way, each BSG and the related factors and events were analyzed independently. The importance of this issue is reflected by the finding that 19 reinterventions for BSGs occurred in 12 patients (1.6 BSG related reinterventions per patient).

NEW STAINLESS STEEL BALLOON EXPANDABLE COVERED STENT

Recently, a new balloon expandable covered received the approval for use in the arterial system. The Gore VBX (Flagstaff, Arizona, US) device has a unique design with stainless steel independent rings. Consequently, the endograft combines flexibility with high radial strength. These features are very important especially in case of angulated aortic side branches optimizing the conformability and apposition of the bridging or chimney device in case of fenestrated or chimney endografting, respectively, in angulated target vessels.

Fig. 17.5 shows a pararenal aneurysm with angulated right renal artery. Fig. 17.6 demonstrates the nice transition and adaption of the distal edge of the VBX in the angulated renal artery. The benefit of this performance is the avoidance of placement of additional flexible nitinol stents minimizing the risk of occlusion due to narrow of the patent lumen in case of placement of more than one covered stents.

SELF-EXPANDING COVERED STENTS

The Gore Viabahn covered stent is a flexible, self-expanding device consisting of an expanded PTFE (ePTFE) lining with an external nitinol support. The new-generation endoprosthesis has four radiopaque markers on each end to improve visibility.

The deployment of the device begins with untwisting the screw-connector at the base of the deployment knob. The preferable deployment technique for the Viabahn is the stepwise placement of the device under

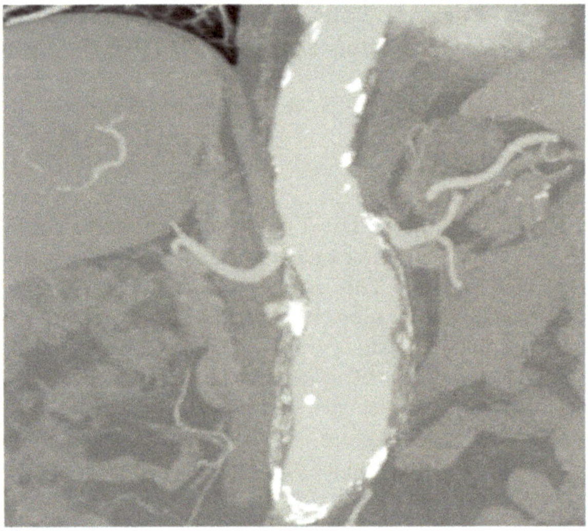

FIG. 17.5 Pararenal aneurysm with angulated renal artery on the right side.

sheath protection (Fig. 17.7). We always stabilize the undeployed segment of the Viabahn with the 7F sheath to avoid full expansion of the device, with the sheath position behind the distal edge of the device. This protects misplacement of the covered stent in angulated target vessels.

The lengths of Viabahn devices used in f/b- and ch-EVAR for juxtarenal aneurysms range between 50 and 100 mm and rarely 150 mm. The devices are compatible with a 7F or 8F sheath with diameters between 5 and 8 mm.

Features

Radial force

Evidence from CTA suggests that the radial force of self-expanding covered stents is lower compared to BECSs. No definitive data exist, however, to compare the radial force of bridging devices in a chimney configuration. Fig. 17.8 presents a chimney case with compression of the Viabahn. The Viabahn is also lined with an additional nitinol bare-metal stent in this case.

Fluoroscopic visibility

The Viabahn device is characterized by poor fluoroscopic visibility. The proximal and distal edge of the device must be visible to ensure an appropriate chimney deployment. A sufficient distal landing zone is adequately visualized only after placement of additional bare-metal stents. This can affect the intraoperative and postoperative outcomes. Use of the newer-generation Viabahn with proximal and distal

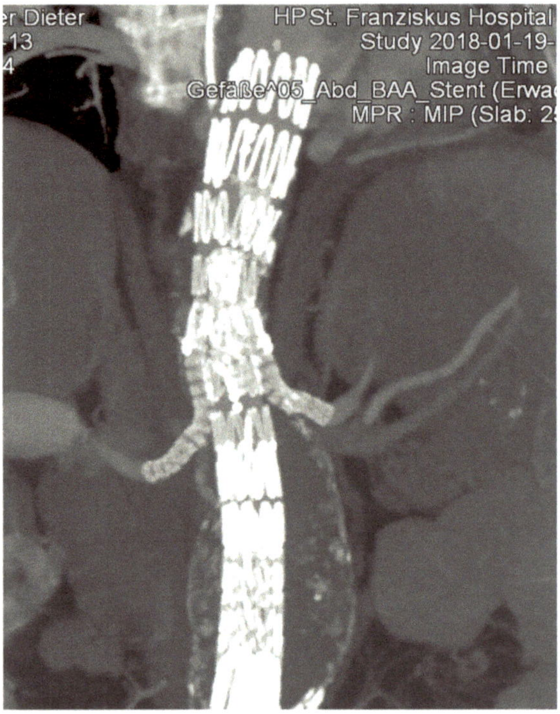

FIG. 17.6 Performance of the VBX covered stent with the flexible distal edge in the angulated renal artery.

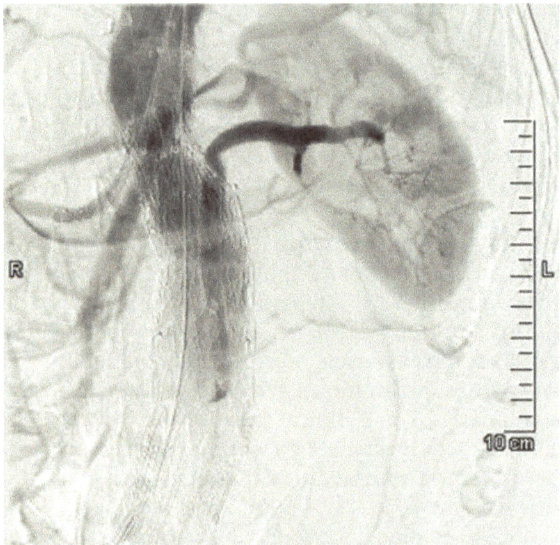

FIG. 17.7 Complete deployment of the Viabahn, with the sheath behind the distal edge of the covered device.

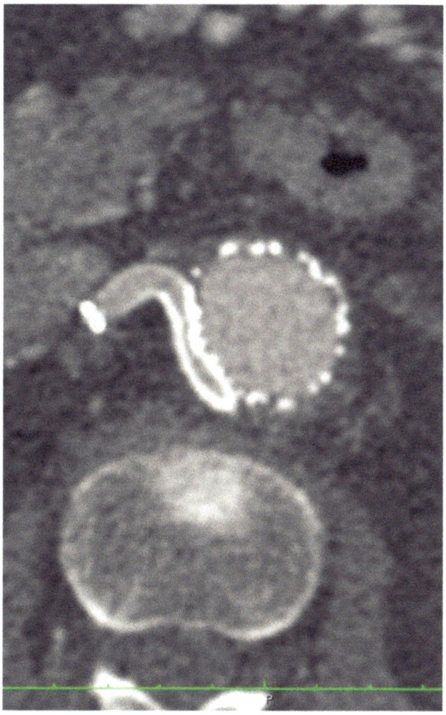

FIG. 17.8 Multiple placements of chimney grafts with use of a nitinol endoskeleton of an abdominal stent-graft, with two balloon-expandable covered stents and one self-expanding covered stent as chimney grafts for the renal arteries and superior mesenteric artery. Note the compression of the proximal edge of the self-expanding device.

markers is likely to overcome this important limitation of the current device.

Flexibility and availability in lengths up to 250 mm

Flexibility of the Viabahn is important in the transfemoral placement of a reversed chimney graft, also known as a *periscope*. Fig. 17.9 shows the placement of a Viabahn from transfemoral access into the left renal artery with type Ia endoleak after previous EVAR. Because of the angulation and need to deploy the device in the distal infrarenal aorta, the flexible and long length (up to 250 mm) of the Viabahn is beneficial.

Literature Review

Extensive literature exists on the use of self-expanding covered stents as chimney devices. A two-arm study compared the performance of self-expanding and balloon-expandable covered stents.[5] Forty-six consecutive target vessels (43 renal, 3 SMA) were revascularized by the Advanta (1.2 chimneys/patient), and 81 consecutive target vessels (64 renal, 11 SMA, 6 celiac trunk) were revascularized by the Viabahn (2.3 chimneys/patient). The success rate for target-vessel preservation was similar: 97.8% for balloon-expandable group and 100% for self-expanding group, on follow-up. Overall, one perioperative (and not present in CTA at discharge) type Ia endoleak was detected in the balloon-expandable group. In contrast, five perioperative type Ia endoleaks were present in the self-expanding group, although only one persisted on postoperative radiologic imaging.

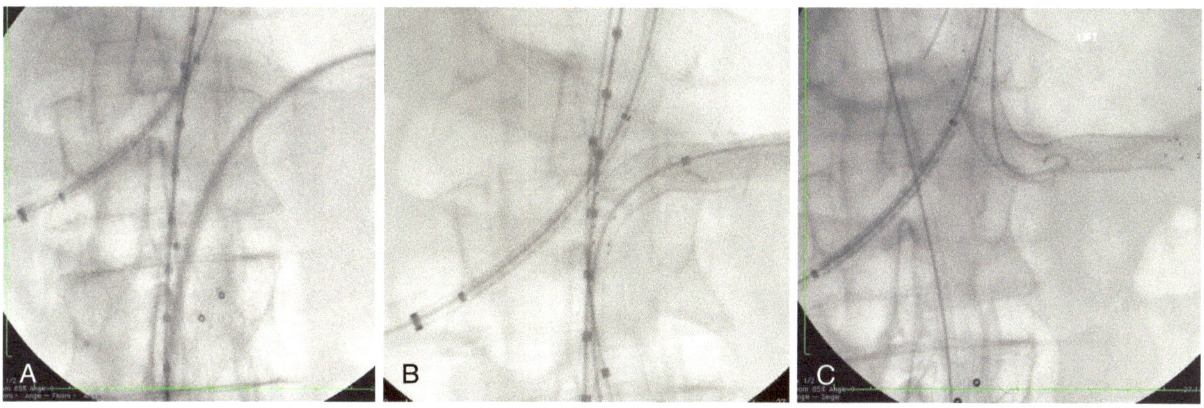

FIG. 17.9 **A-C,** Demonstration of the lift technique by chimney endografting. A Viabahn was deployed from the transfemoral access in the left renal artery. Additionally, the distal edge of the Viabahn will be fixed by placement of a short balloon. Finally, the proximal edge was moved cranially by the 8F sheath from transfemoral access.

This patient was treated with a proximal extension of a 5-mm cuff 1 year postoperatively because of aneurysm sac enlargement.

In summary, midterm results of covered chimney stents used for pararenal aortic pathologies confirmed their safety and feasibility, with excellent patency and a low incidence of endoleaks, regardless of whether balloon-expandable or self-expanding covered stents were used.

In agreement with this experience, the Zurich group published the performance of 169 revascularized branches with chimney/periscope grafts (CPGs), followed for 2 years. Overall, four CPGs occluded (98% target-vessel patency); no stent-graft migration was observed. Renal function remained stable in all patients.[6]

Lining

The concept of lining consists of placement of nitinol self-expanding bare-metal stents outside the distal edge of the previously deployed covered stents, to achieve a smooth transition of the chimney graft in angulated target vessels. Also, this configuration creates a funnel shape, potentially reducing the risk for the development of hyperplasia and stenosis or occlusion of the bridging stent.

REFERENCES

1. Donas KP, Lee JT, Lachat M, et al. Collected world experience about the performance of the snorkel/chimney endovascular technique in the treatment of complex aortic pathologies: the PERICLES Registry. *Ann Surg*. 2015;262(3):53–546: discussion 552–553.
2. Donas KP, Torsello GB, Piccoli G, et al. The PROTAGORAS study to evaluate the performance of the Endurant stent graft for patients with pararenal pathologic processes treated by the chimney/snorkel endovascular technique. *J Vasc Surg*. 2016;63(1):1–7.
3. Panuccio G, Bisdas T, Berekoven B, Torsello G, Austermann M. Performance of bridging stent grafts in fenestrated and branched aortic endografting. *Eur J Vasc Endovasc Surg*. 2015;50(1):60–70.
4. Mastracci TM, Greenberg RK, Eagleton MJ, Hernandez AV. Durability of branches in branched and fenestrated endografts. *J Vasc Surg*. 2013;57(4):926–933.
5. Donas KP, Pecoraro F, Torsello G, et al. Use of covered chimney stents for pararenal aortic pathologies is safe and feasible with excellent patency and low incidence of endoleaks. *J Vasc Surg*. 2012;55(3):659–665.
6. Lachat M, Veith FJ, Pfammatter T, et al. Chimney and periscope grafts observed over 2 years after their use to revascularize 169 renovisceral branches in 77 patients with complex aortic aneurysms. *J Endovasc Ther*. 2013;20(5):597–605. https://doi.org/10.1583/13-4372.1.

CHAPTER 18

Management of Type Ia Endoleaks

KONSTANTINOS P. DONAS • GIOVANNI TORSELLO

Use of endovascular techniques in the treatment of abdominal aortic aneurysms (AAAs) was revolutionary. Less invasive approaches and improved endovascular equipment led to expanded treatment of AAAs in technically demanding anatomies. At the same time, however, late complications such as type I endoleaks have increasingly occurred.

A primary reason for type Ia endoleaks after endovascular aneurysm repair (EVAR) is an undersized, previously deployed endograft, with insufficient apposition and fixation with the aortic wall. In this case, optimization of the fixation with EndonAchors or balloon-expandable stents, or administration of fluid agents in the gap between the device and the aortic wall, should be considered. EndoAnchors (Aptus Endosystems, Sunnyvale, California) or Palmaz bare-metal stents (Cordis, Fremont, California) can be an option only in the case of neck enlargement without significant migration of the previous endograft. The Aneurysm Treatment using the Heli-FX Aortic Securement System Global Registry (ANCHOR) demonstrated high technical success of 95% in 319 patients, but also 9.1% residual type Ia endoleak at the end of the procedure.[1]

Regarding the use of Palmaz stents, a retrospective review from the Cleveland Clinic (Ohio, USA) showed primary reported technical success of 100%.[2] However, in 35% of the treated cases, the authors observed mid-term loss of the proximal seal zone and adaptation of the Palmaz stent with the aortic stent-graft and wall. Major limitations of the Palmaz stents are the rigidity and inability of the device to follow the natural neck enlargement, which can lead to new type Ia endoleak.

A common reason for the majority of the migrated endografts is severe aortic neck angulation, which provokes stent-graft migration and partial occlusion of the origin of the renal arteries from the struts of the suprarenal bare-metal stent. In this particular case, creation of new sealing zone is the recommended approach. This can be accomplished by using fenestrated endografts.

Katsargyris et al.[3] reported one of the largest series in the literature regarding treatment of 26 patients by fenestrated EVAR. The authors confirm the technical difficulty of catheterizing the renal ostia through the fenestrations in 23.1% of the treated cases, with the struts of the suprarenal stent between the target vessels and the fenestrations. In addition, in five patients (19.2%), iliac access through the previous stent graft was tedious and caused some dislodgment of the preexisting stent-graft and alterations in the available working length. In agreement with the Nurnberg experience, the Cleveland Clinic reported that branched and fenestrated repair after failed EVAR is more complex than repair in the native aorta.[4]

In contrast to fenestrated endografts, use of parallel grafts has some clear advantages. First, using off-the-shelf devices permits immediate treatment without delay. This is important for these rupture-threatening pathologic processes; in the experience of our cohort, the median aortic diameter of the treated cases was 7.1 cm.[5]

From a technical point of view, catheterization from the upper extremity in a normally downward-oriented target vessel is easier and feasible. In addition, use of Endurant tubes with the short, M-shaped stents allows harmonic adaptability of the device in angulated necks, leading to successful exclusion of the pathologic process. At the same time, the low-profile introducer system allows trackability of severe iliac calcifications and angulations. Finally, placement of the abdominal device by chimney-graft EVAR follows insertion and positioning of the sheaths in the target vessels. In the event of unsuccessful catheterization of the target vessels, interruption of the intervention is always possible. In contrast, inability to catheterize the target vessels through the fenestrations after placement of a fenestrated endograft will lead to surgical conversion and explantation of the fenestrated endograft. This may be associated with a high-risk patient who is unfit for open repair, with profound clinical complications.

On the other hand, a major issue with the chimney technique remains the ideal combination of chimney and abdominal grafts to minimize the risk for persistent gutters. Based on our advanced experience with parallel and fenestrated grafts, use of balloon-expandable covered stents in the renovisceral target vessels has clear benefits regarding fluoroscopic visibility, precise positioning, and radial force.

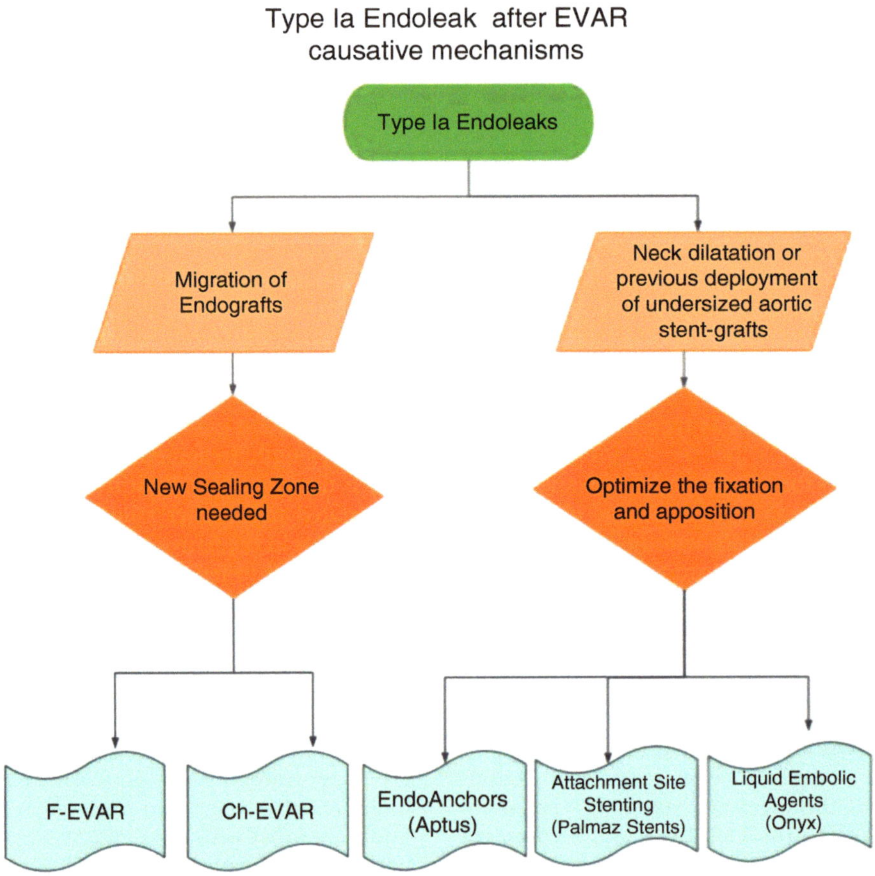

FIG. 18.1 Causative mechanisms and therapeutic techniques and devices for type Ia endoleaks after endovascular aneurysm repair (EVAR). *F-EVAR*, Fenestrated EVAR; *Ch-EVAR*, chimney-graft EVAR.

In one patient, we observed a contained rupture caused by gutter-associated endoleak, demonstrating the substantial need for meticulous follow-up.[5] The patient was treated successfully by endovascular means, with no need for surgical conversion. In this case we used a sandwich configuration with a migrated Zenith device, the periscope Viabahn graft from transfemoral access because of inability to catheterize the left renal artery from the upper extremity, and finally Endurant tubes from outward to inward. One possible explanation of the persistent and unplanned created gutters is the inappropriate interaction of the flexible Viabahn periscope graft with the rigid, stainless steel endoskeleton of the Zenith device.

Fig. 18.1 presents the treatment algorithm of type Ia endoleaks after EVAR based on the causative mechanisms. Clinical data are needed to establish the presented approach.

REFERENCES

1. Jordan WD, Mehta M, Varnagy D, et al. Results of the ANCHOR prospective, multicenter registry of EndoAnchors for type Ia endoleaks and endograft migration in patients with challenging anatomy. *J Vasc Surg*. 2014;60:885–892.
2. Arthurs ZM, Lyden SP, Rajani RR, Eagleton MJ, Clair DG. Long-term outcomes of Palmaz stent placement for intraoperative type Ia endoleak during endovascular aneurysm repair. *Ann Vasc Surg*. 2011;25:120–126.
3. Katsargyris A, Yazar O, Oikonomou K, et al. Fenestrated stent-grafts for salvage of prior endovascular abdominal aortic aneurysm repair. *Eur J Vasc Endovasc Surg*. 2013;46:49–56.
4. Martin Z, Greenberg RK, Mastracci TM, Eagleton MJ, O'Callaghan A, Bena J. Late rescue of proximal endograft failure using fenestrated and branched devices. *J Vasc Surg*. 2014;59:1479–1487.
5. Donas KP, Telve D, Torsello G, Pitoulias G, Schwindt A, Austermann M. Use of parallel grafts to save failed prior endovascular aortic aneurysm repair and type Ia endoleaks. *J Vasc Surg*. 2015;62(3):578–584.

Management of Type II Endoleaks with Ethylene-Vinyl-Alcohol Copolymer Liquid Embolic Agent

KONSTANTINOS P. DONAS • MICHEL BOSIERS • ARNE SCHWINDT

Treatment of abdominal aortic aneurysms (AAAs) has evolved significantly during the last two decades, especially with the broader introduction of endovascular aneurysm repair (EVAR) by Parodi et al.[1] in 1991. However, the Achilles' heel of EVAR remains the endoleak.

Many early type II endoleaks are transient and will resolve spontaneously within 6 months with conservative treatment alone. When a type II endoleak is associated with aneurysm sac enlargement of more than 5 mm, however, treatment of the endoleak is necessary.[2-5] Different treatment options have been described, including embolization through a transarterial, lumbar (direct puncture), and caval route; laparoscopic ligation; and open surgical repair. Onyx is an embolic agent approved by the U.S. Food and Drug Administration (FDA) for the embolization of arteriovenous malformations in the brain. A similar predecessor compound was first described in the early 1990s by Taki et al.[6] and Terada et al.[7].

Onyx is an ethylene-vinyl-alcohol copolymer (EVOH) dissolved in dimethyl sulfoxide (DMSO) and suspended micronized tantalum powder (Medtronic, Santa Rosa, California, USA). There are three possible concentrations:

- Onyx LES (liquid embolic system) 18 (6% EVOH)
- Onyx LES 34 (8% EVOH)
- Onyx HD 500 (20% EVOH)

The greater the amount of copolymer, the higher the viscosity. Solidification takes place within 5 minutes after injection.

PREOPERATIVE EVALUATION

Multislice (1.0-mm) computed tomography angiography (CTA) with arterial and venous phases is performed to define the endoleak anatomically. Inflow from two main sources is responsible for the development and persistence of type II endoleaks:

1. Flow into the aneurysm sac from the inferior mesenteric artery (IMA) via the Riolan anastomosis and the superior mesenteric artery (SMA)
2. Lumbar or middle sacral artery inflow originating from the hypogastric artery and via the iliolumbar artery to the feeding branch vessels

Combined inflow from both the IMA and the lumbar vessels can also occur.

Once the location of the vessels feeding and draining a type II endoleak is confirmed, transarterial embolization with Onyx is our preferred approach in Münster, Germany. Fig. 19.1 shows CTA of a patient with type II endoleak originating from the IMA.

When no inflow vessels are detected, or a transarterial attempt fails, a translumbar approach becomes the therapy of choice. Ultimately, if endovascular treatment of a type II endoleak fails, continued aneurysm enlargement dictates a more invasive therapy, such as open surgical repair (Fig. 19.2).

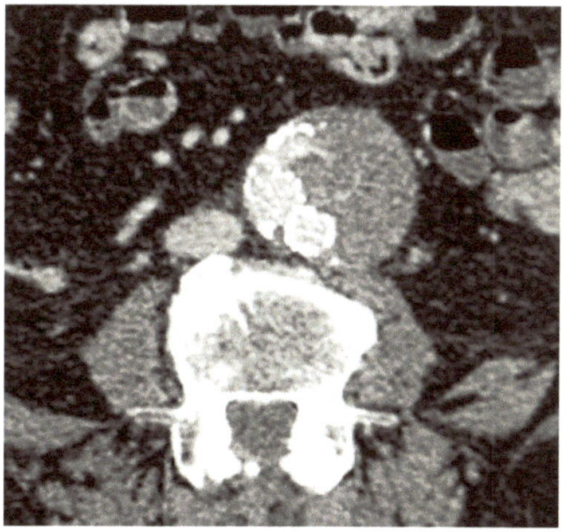

FIG. 19.1 Type II endoleak originating from inferior mesenteric artery leading to an increase of the aneurysm sac.

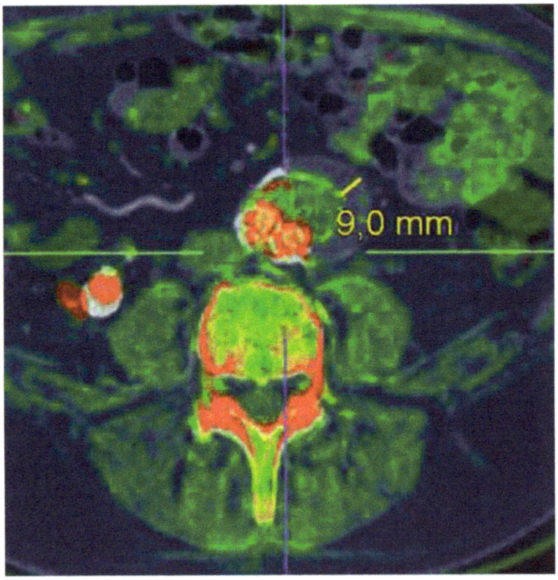

FIG. 19.2 Fusion of two postoperative CTA scans shows significant enlargement of the aneurysm sac of 9 mm in 8 months.

SURGICAL APPROACH

Onyx embolization can be performed through brachial or common femoral artery access. We prefer the transbrachial approach, to avoid a 180-degree orientation of the sheath and catheter in relationship to the iliolumbar artery through the ipsilateral internal iliac artery with transfemoral access. If the patient is very tall, a transaxillary approach is mandatory to have enough catheter length to reach the iliolumbar artery. We perform the procedure usually with the patient under general anesthesia.

PROCEDURE

- The left brachial artery is punctured and a short, 4-French (4F) sheath introduced using Seldinger technique.
- Heparin (5000 IU) is administered.
- A 0.035-inch, soft Terumo wire is advanced into the ascending aorta. After rotation of the pigtail catheter and on rapid advancement of the wire, the catheter can be easily advanced into the renovisceral aortic segment.
- Over a stiff wire, a 6F Shuttle sheath of 90 cm (Cook, Bloomington, Indiana, USA) is placed in the renovisceral aortic portion.
- With a soft wire and a vertebral catheter, the SMA is cannulated (Fig. 19.3). After identification of the Riolan anastomosis (Fig. 19.4), both the sheath and the vertebral catheter are advanced as far as possible.

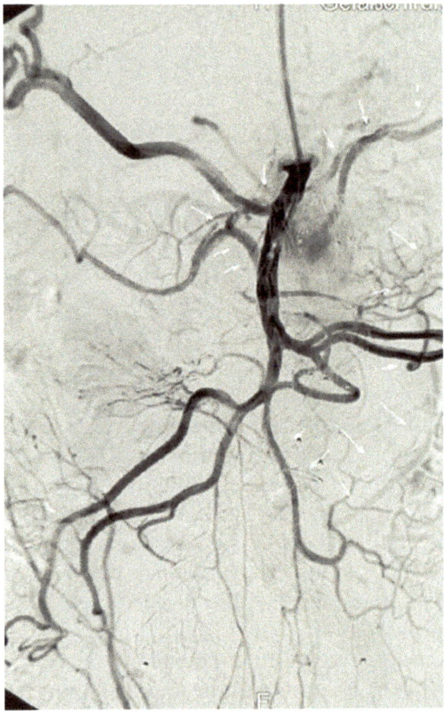

FIG. 19.3 Superselective angiography of the superior mesenteric artery.

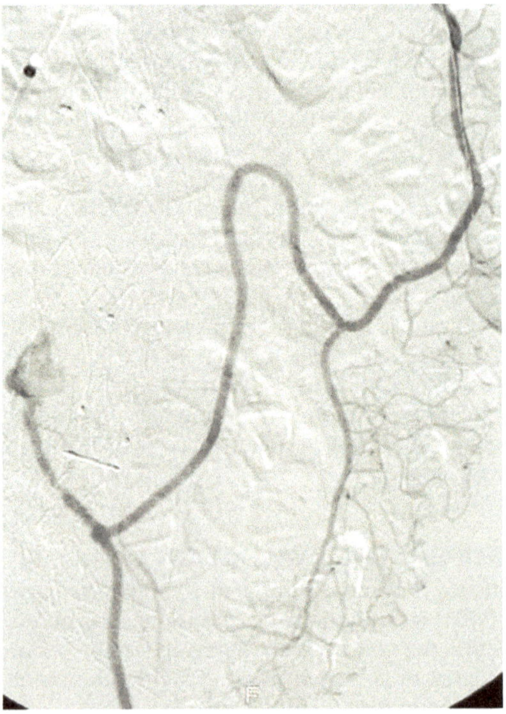

FIG. 19.4 Example of the Riolan anastomosis and its connection with the inferior mesenteric artery.

- When the endoleak originates from the lumbar arteries, the internal iliac artery is entered, followed by cannulation of the iliolumbar artery. Through a vertebral catheter, a 0.014-inch wire is advanced into the endoleak cavity.
- The endoleak is now entered with DMSO-compatible microcatheters, such as the 0.014-inch Echelon or 0.010-inch Marathon (Medtronic).
- In preparation for Onyx embolization, the microcatheter is flushed with saline and then prepared with DMSO to fill the dead space in order to prevent premature polymerization of Onyx, since it polymerizes from contact with water or blood. The goal of embolization is to occlude the endoleak nidus and both the inflow and the outflow vessels (Fig. 19.5). Onyx is deployed into the feeding vessel during withdrawal of the catheter.
- The injection of Onyx concludes when the outflow vessels start to fill up with Onyx (Fig. 19.6). The catheter then is carefully retracted under aspiration of the Onyx syringe.

Fig. 19.7 shows the postoperative imaging. In this case, we used magnetic resonance imaging (MRI). With CT there is always artifact from the tantalum powder, although it provides the necessary radiopacity for the controlled fluoroscopic delivery.

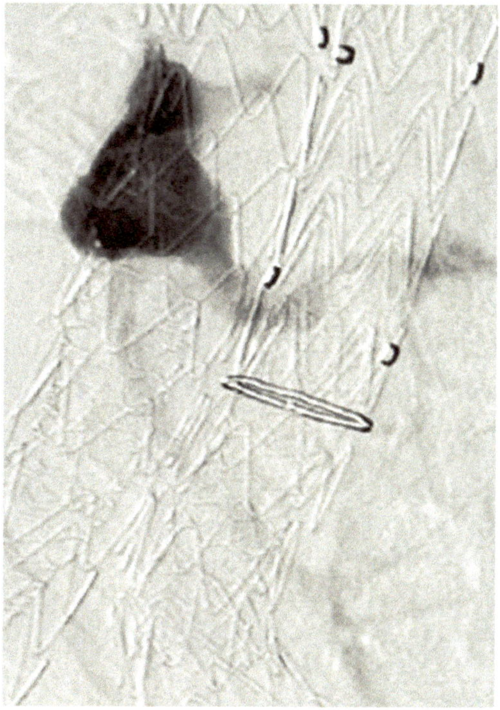

FIG. 19.5 The endoleak nidus.

LITERATURE REVIEW

Bosiers et al.[8] reported the use of Onyx in 13 patients with persistent type II endoleaks leading to aneurysm sac growth greater than 5 mm in diameter. Transarterial Onyx embolization was performed in each case, with technical success of 92% (12 of 13 patients). In one patient, repeated efforts to cannulate the target vessel responsible for the endoleak led to a rupture of the hypogastric artery; which was treated by covered stent implantation. Clinical success was 90% (9 of 10 patients).

In 2000, Martin et al.[9] reported on complete endoleak obliteration in five of six patients treated with Onyx. A left-sided translumbar puncture was used in three patients, transcaval puncture in one patient, and IMA catheterization in two patients. Follow-up imaging demonstrated decreased aneurysm diameter in all patients at 7 to 29 weeks (mean, 19.2 weeks) after treatment. Simpson et al.[10] used translumbar embolization exclusively to treat type II endoleaks, with a success rate of only 45.5% (5 of 11 patients).

Baum et al.[11] showed a significant advantage of the translumbar access over a transarterial embolization

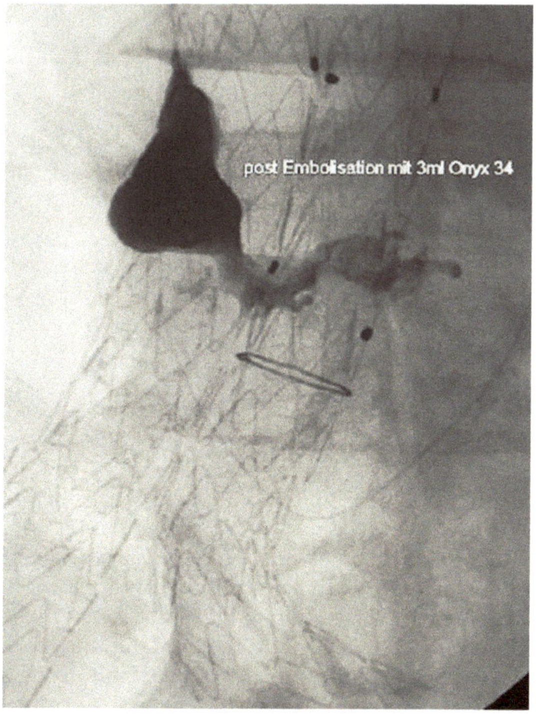

FIG. 19.6 Treatment result after Onyx embolization.

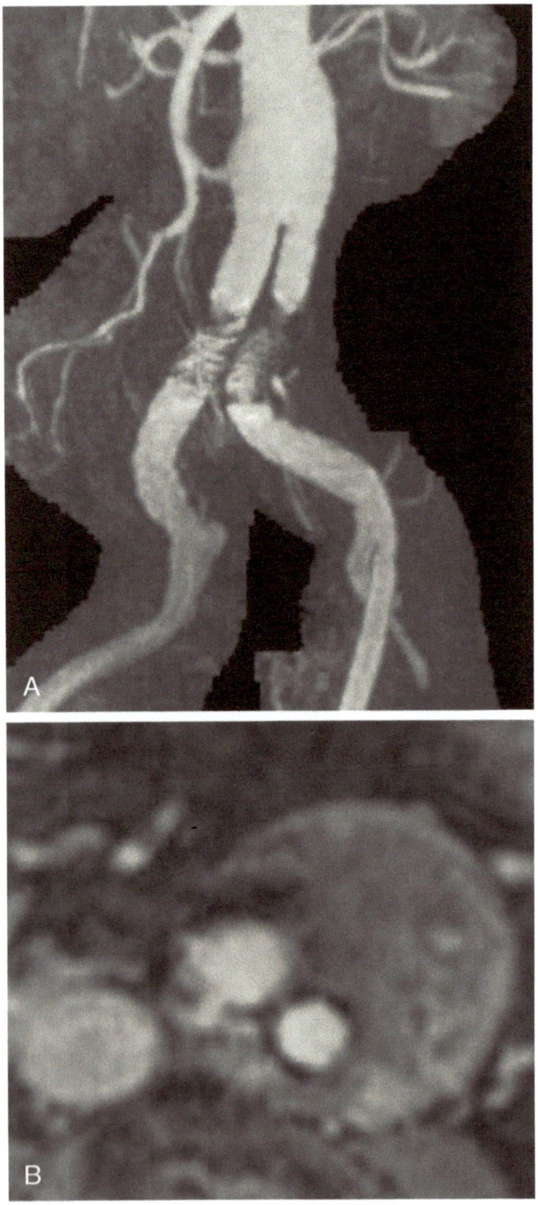

FIG. 19.7 **A, B,** Postoperative imaging after Onyx embolization.

technique. Stavropoulos et al.[12] provided an explanation for this difference, with coils directly deployed into the endoleak cavity closing the nidus of the feeding vessel. In the Baum study, coils were deployed into the feeding vessel itself, leaving the nidus untreated. Embolizing the nidus achieves more consistent outcome than coiling a single feeding vessel.

ADVANTAGES AND DISADVANTAGES

N-butyl cyanoacrylate (NBC) and Onyx were described as liquid embolic agents. Comparing both agents, Onyx has several advantages.[13] Onyx is resistant to adherence to the delivery catheter, allowing a slower, more controlled delivery. Further, the risk of injury to the target lesion is minimized when the catheter is removed. The controlled delivery also minimizes inadvertent distal embolization to a nontarget location. In this regard, mesenteric ischemia and paraparesis have been described as complications caused by distal migration of NBC.[13,14] Because of the difference in solidification and the ability to inject over a longer period, a higher volume of Onyx can be deployed per session.

Disadvantages of Onyx include the preparation time, transient halitosis and unpleasant body odor, high costs, and potential for vasospasm.[15,16] Although minimized, the risk of end-organ ischemia remains when Onyx is not carefully deployed. Also, Onyx causes CT artifact from the tantalum powder necessary to provide radiopacity for the controlled delivery. Therefore, we recommend magnetic resonance angiography (MRA) for an accurate measurement of the aneurysm sac after Onyx treatment.

REFERENCES

1. Parodi JC, Palmaz JC, Barone HD. Transfemoral intraluminal graft implantation for abdominal aortic aneurysms. *Ann Vasc Surg*. 1991;5:491–499.
2. Schlösser FJ, Gusberg RJ, Dardik A, et al. Aneurysm rupture after EVAR: can the ultimate failure be predicted? *Eur J Vasc Endovasc Surg*. 2009;37:15–22.
3. Van Marrewijk CJ, Fransen G, Laheij RJ, Harris PL, Buth J. Is a type II endoleak after EVAR a harbringer of risk? Causes and outcome of open conversion and aneurysm rupture during follow-up. *Eur J Vasc Endovasc Surg*. 2004;27:128–137.
4. Jones JE, Atkins MD, Brewster DC, et al. Persistent type II endoleak after endovascular repair of abdominal aortic aneurysm is associated with adverse late outcomes. *J Vasc Surg*. 2007;46:1–8.
5. Higashiura W, Greenberg RK, Katz E, Geiger L, Bathhurst S. Predictive factors, morphologic effects and proposed treatment paradigm for type II endoleaks after repair of infrarenal abdominal aortic aneurysms. *J Vasc Interv Radiol*. 2007;18:875–881.
6. Taki W, Yonekawa Y, Iwata H, uno A, Yamashita K, Amemiya H. A new liquid material for embolization of arteriovenous malformations. *AJNR Am J Neuroradiol*. 1990;11:163–168.
7. Terada T, Nakamura Y, Nakai K, et al. Embolization of arteriovenous malformations with peripheral aneurysms using ethylene vinyl alcohol copolymer: report of three cases. *J Neurosurg*. 1991;75:655–660.

8. Bosiers MJ, Schwindt A, Donas KP, Torsello G. Midterm results of the transarterial use of Onyx in the treatment of persisting type II endoleaks after EVAR. *J Cardiovasc Surg*. 2013;54(4):469–475.
9. Martin ML, Dolmatch BL, Fry PD, Machan LS. Treatment of type II endoleaks with Onyx. *J Vasc Interv Radiol*. 2001;12:629–632.
10. Simpson AJ, Garg J, Dilley RB, Frankel D, Kansal N. Translumbar embolization of for type II endoleaks after EVAR: a multicenter retrospective review. *J Vasc Surg*. 2010;52(2):529.
11. Baum RA, Carpenter JP, Golden MA, et al. Treatment of type 2 endoleaks after endovascular repair of abdominal aortic aneurysms: comparison of transarterial and translumbar techniques. *J Vasc Surg*. 2002;35:23–29.
12. Stavropoulos SW, Park J, Fairman R, Carpenter J. Type 2 endoleak embolization comparison: translumbar embolization versus modified transarterial embolization. *J Vasc Interv Radiol*. 2009;20(10):1299–1302.
13. Massis K, Carson 3rd WG, Rozas A, Patel V, Zwiebel B. Treatment of type II endoleaks with ethylene-vinyl-alcohol copolymer (Onyx). *Vasc Endovascular Surg*. 2012;46(3): 251–257.
14. Abularrage CJ, Patel VI, Conrad MF, Schneider EB, Cambria RP, Kwolek CJ. Improved results using Onyx glue for the treatment of persistent type 2 endoleak after endovascular aneurysm repair. *J Vasc Surg*. 2012;56(3):630–636. Epub 2012 May 8.
15. Chao CP, Paz-Fumagalli R, Walser EM, et al. Percutaneous protective coil occlusion of the proximal inferior mesenteric artery before *N*-butyl cyanoacrylate embolization of type II endoleaks after endovascular repair of abdominal aortic aneurysms. *J Vasc Interv Radiol*. 2006;17:1827–1833.
16. Gambaro E, Abou-Zamzam Jr AM, Teruya TH, Bianchi C, Hopewell J, Ballard JL. Ischemic colitis following translumbar thrombin injection for treatment of endoleak. *Ann Vasc Surg*. 2004;18(1):74–78.

CHAPTER 20

Fusion Techniques in Advanced Endovascular Repair

GIUSEPPE PANUCCIO • GIOVANNI FEDERICO TORSELLO • JOHANNES SCHÄFERS • KONSTANTINOS P. DONAS • GIOVANNI TORSELLO

The performance of increasingly complex endovascular procedures has prompted a need for more eloquent angiographic imaging at the time of the initial procedure The amount of ionizing radiation and contrast media is directly proportional to the complexity of the procedure.

To reduce radiation and contrast dose, the intraoperative use of fusion technologies during endovascular aneurysm repair (EVAR) and fenestrated/branched EVAR (f/b-EVAR) was introduced by the Cleveland Clinic group in 2010.[1] The technique comprises a combination of preoperative computed tomography angiography (CTA) with conventional intraprocedural angiographic techniques.

The technology allows the merging of precise CT-based three-dimensional (3D) anatomic information with the two-dimensional (2D) dynamic functional imaging based on intraoperative fluoroscopy. Fusion imaging provides the complementary benefit of both imaging systems, achieving a reduction of the radiation exposure and contrast dose normally required in such procedures.

INDICATIONS

Fusion overlay imaging can be used for every endovascular procedure if a preoperative CTA or magnetic resonance angiography (MRA) scan has been obtained. The greatest advantage is when target vessels need to be cannulated. The use of fusion imaging is especially attractive for advanced endovascular aortic repair. It also helps to overcome challenging anatomies with angulated aortic necks, tortuous vessels, and accessory aortic branches. The application of the technique can simplify complex aortic procedures, decrease the duration of the interventional procedure, and lower radiation exposure.

TECHNIQUE

Currently, the latest-generation hybrid operating room (OR) is equipped with advanced imaging tools such as fusion imaging. These are coupled with a workstation to load and process the DICOM (Digital Imaging and Communications in Medicine) data from a previous CT (or less frequently MR) scan. A 3D model of the vasculature is segmented and then merged with the live fluoroscopic image. Several imaging companies have developed radio-proprietary systems to combine the different technologies. Recently, Cyder Medica developed a new system able to integrate the required workstation for the fusion technology in every OR angiographic system, including mobile C-arm equipment.

Prerequisites to fusion imaging are (1) the ability to extrapolate vessel anatomy from the 3D DICOM dataset, (2) a precise registration system of the image modalities, and (3) the ability to select and show the operator the relevant aspect of the patient anatomy on the live image without impairing the image quality.

The technique is performed in four simple, automated and manually assisted steps: (1) segmentation, (2) planning, (3) registration, and (4) live image guidance.

Segmentation

At first, the DICOM dataset from the preoperative CT or MR scan is loaded into the workstation. The anatomic structure pertinent to the procedure is selected, limiting the view to the relevant vasculature. Most of the available segmentation engines work semiautomatically. With a point-and-click system, the vessels of interest are selected for further processing (e.g., abdominal aorta and renal, iliac, and hypogastric arteries for infrarenal EVAR) (Fig. 20.1).

Planning

For detailed planning of the procedure, the software allows the operator to set *markers* on vessel origins and *rings* orthogonal to the vessel. The markers and rings can be adjusted in all three axes and named, measured, and applied with captions (Fig. 20.2).

This step helps to visualize landing zones and provides cannulation guidance. Furthermore, it aids in planning the optimal angles and parallax for intraoperative angiography and deployment of devices (Fig. 20.3).

Recently, another fully automatic system has been introduced that not only performs segmentation of the entire aorta and main branches (Fig. 20.4A, *red structure*), but also creates a mathematical representation of the vessels, highlighting the takeoff (Fig. 20.4B, *blue rings*), length of the vessels (*graduated center green line*), and best projection of each vessel (*yellow rings*).

Registration

This step aligns the "fusion" of preoperative slice imaging (CT or MR scan) to the real-time fluoroscopic image in the angiosuite. Two modalities are currently available to obtain a correct overlapping of the two datasets: 3D/3D and 2D/3D registration.

3D/3D registration

The initial 3D/3D registration method requires the intraoperative acquisition of a volume dataset of the patient's anatomy. This can be performed with new, fixed angiography systems that can perform a cone-beam CT. Through an almost complete rotation of the C-arm around the area of interest, it is possible to obtain a CT in the angiosuite (Fig. 20.5A, *left*).

The acquisition takes approximately 10 seconds, and if needed, contrast can be injected. After this process, the volume dataset coming from the preoperative CT scan must be combined with the intraoperative 3D dataset. An accurate alignment between the two datasets requires a manual matching process of the anatomic region, which can be cumbersome and prolonged. It involves several potentially error-prone steps, where inaccuracies can occur because the

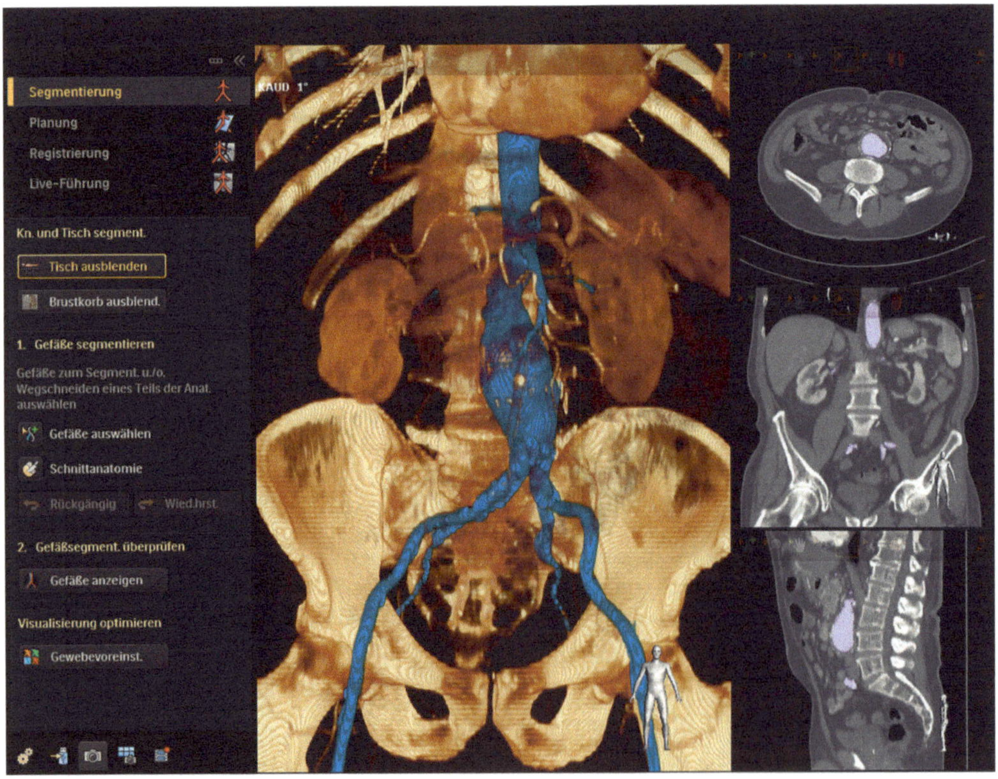

FIG. 20.1 The aorta as well as the renal arteries and iliac vessels have been selected (*blue*) to be visualized in the intraoperative phases.

registration technique relies purely on the patient's position at the moment of the two acquisitions. Further, in the event of patient movement, an additional cone-beam CT scan is needed to correct the misalignment. Recently, Philips (Andover, Massachusetts, USA) introduced a semiautomatic method to facilitate this process. The operator marks three points on different slices in the preoperative- and intraoperative volume data. A registration is then performed on calculations based on these three landmarks (Fig. 20.5A, B).

Briefly, major limitations are the need for additional radiation dose and the risk of contaminating the surgical field from the required rotational movement of the C-arm.

2D/3D registration

In 2D/3D registration an intraoperative 2D dataset is matched with the preoperative 3D dataset. The 3D data of the CT scan is merged with a 2D fluoroscopic image in the angiosuite. At least two projections in different angulations need to be performed. Some systems require only bone structures as markers, and no additional contrast agent is needed; others also combine the visualization of the vessels. The merging is achieved by matching bony landmarks of two single 2D images with the bones in the CT scan. The two images should include an anterior-posterior and an angled left (LAO) or right (RAO) anterior oblique projection of 45 to 90 degrees.

Normally, a 3D segmentation of the vessels and bones is overlapped with the two projections, and the operator is required to translate and rotate the 3D volume dataset along the three axes of the space to obtain a perfect matching of the structures (Fig. 20.6). Most often, the vertebral bodies and the iliac crests are matched in these 2D projections with the 3D dataset of the preoperative scan. This step is performed manually at the workstation and normally takes a few minutes.

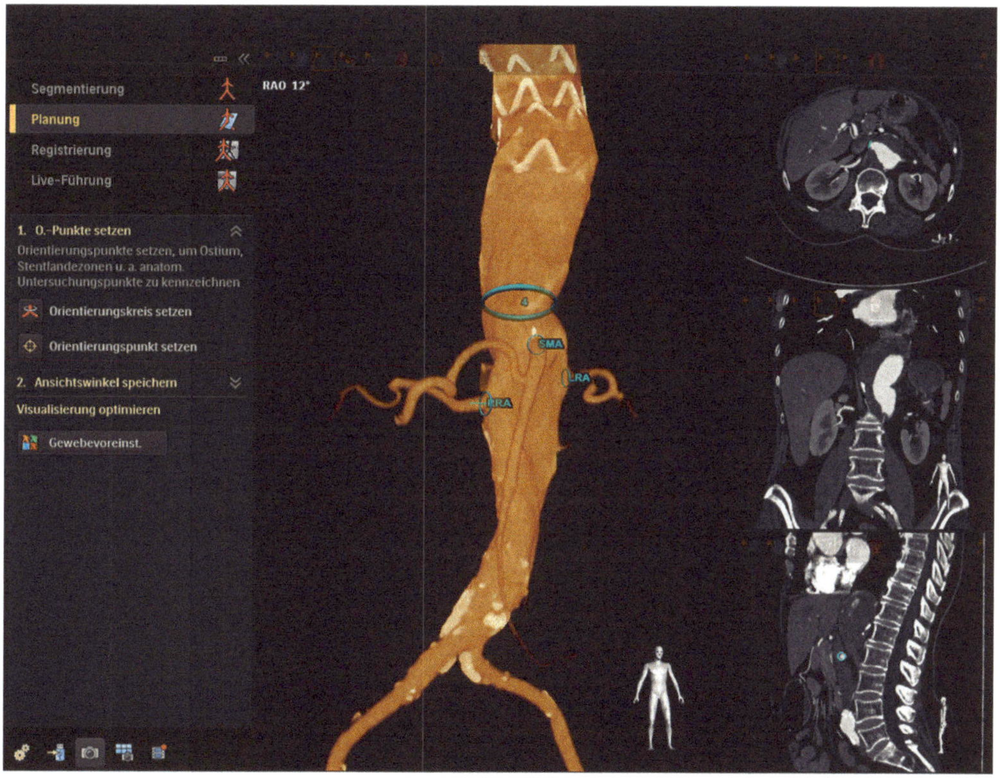

A

FIG. 20.2 **A,** Aneurysm degeneration in the thoracoabdominal segment.

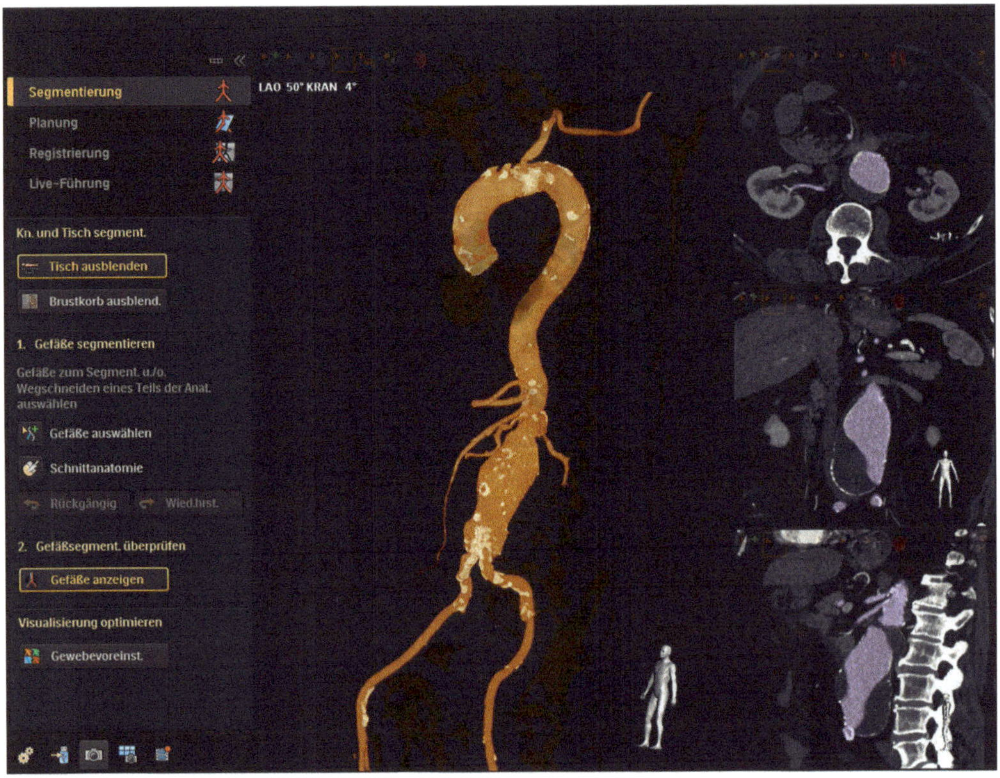

B

FIG. 20.2, cont'd B, Takeoffs of the superior mesenteric artery (SMA) and the left and right renal artery (LRA and RRA) are marked with a small blue ring. An additional ring (number 4) is placed to indicate the best projection of the aorta.

The process can be repeated each time a misalignment is noted. However, vessel deformation, such as that related to the use of stiff wires, can be a source of misalignment (Fig. 20.7). To overcome this problem, Siemens (Erlangen, Germany) introduced an automated calculation able to verify the correct matching in different projections and eventually modify the vessel anatomy according to the device.

Live Image Guidance

After successful registration, the alignment is locked, and the 3D overlay image is visualized on the fluoroscopic image intraoperatively. Different visualizations of the 3D overlay image can be selected to fit the situation and the operator's needs. This can be a 3D mesh model, with a solid or discontinuous lumen outline (Fig. 20.8). In addition, the markers and rings defined in the planning step are visualized three-dimensionally (Figs. 20.9 and 20.10).

LITERATURE REVIEW

Since its introduction, several studies have shown the feasibility of the fusion technique and its advantages in complex aortic procedures. The applicability of the Siemens automated fusion imaging engine has been reported with a high success rate and low deviation from the overlay mesh model.[2] The fusion technology has significantly reduced the use of contrast medium during f/b-EVAR and resulted in shorter procedure times.[3] The Lille group observed that use of the fusion technique in standard and complex EVAR resulted in a reduction of radiation doses for both patients and operators.[4]

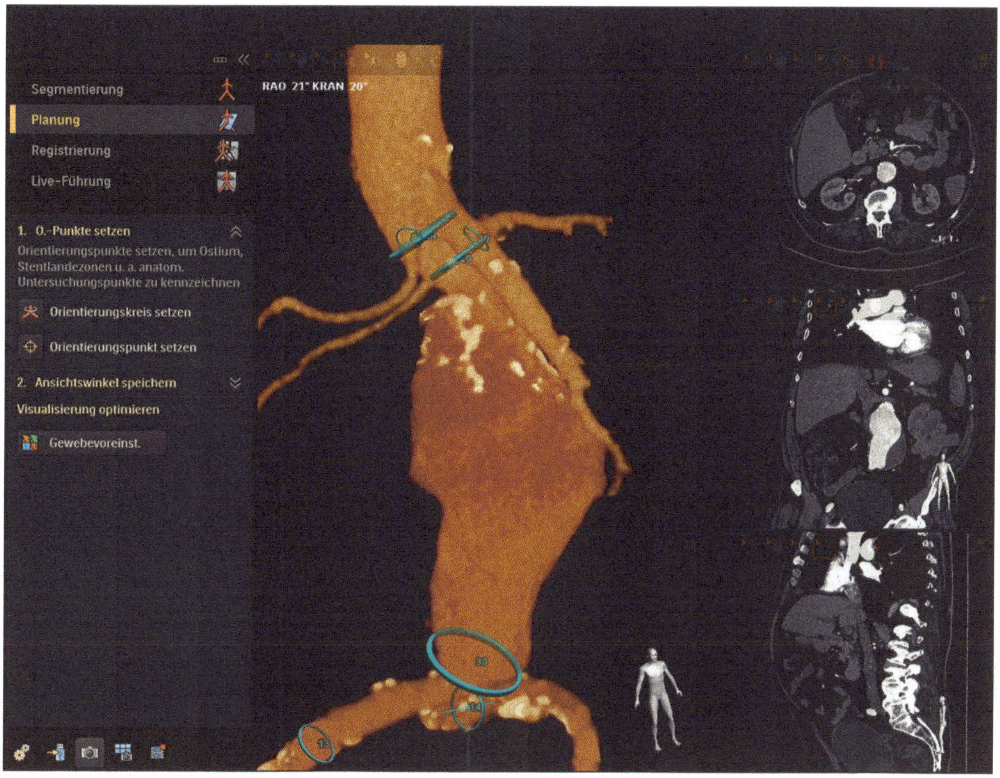

FIG. 20.3 Pararenal aortic aneurysm. The choice of the best working projection is a key step of each endovascular procedure. In this case, the ring at the level of the proximal aortic neck is visualized as a line, indicating the absence of parallax.

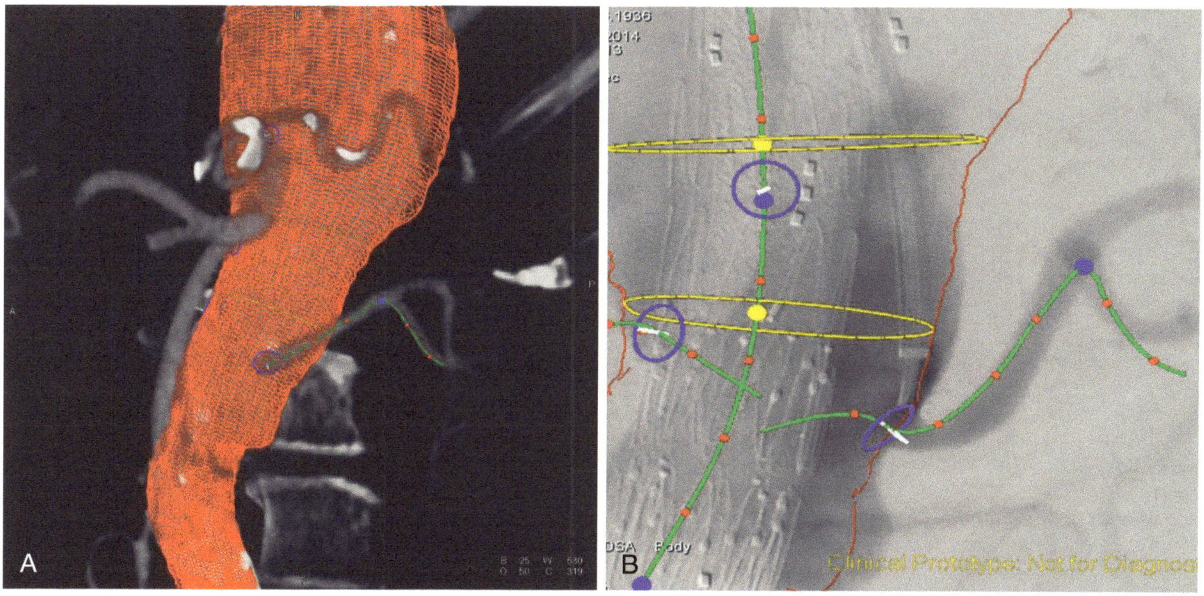

FIG. 20.4 **A,** Mathematical representation of a thoracoabdominal aortic aneurysm. The *red network* is automatically reconstructed following the aortic lumen. **B,** Detail of intraoperative fluoroscopy with merged mesh model. *Blue rings* are placed at the level of the main side vessels. A *green line* depicts the centerline of the vessel, and *red points* are placed along the line at each centimeter. The *yellow rings* show the orientation of the aortic lumen.

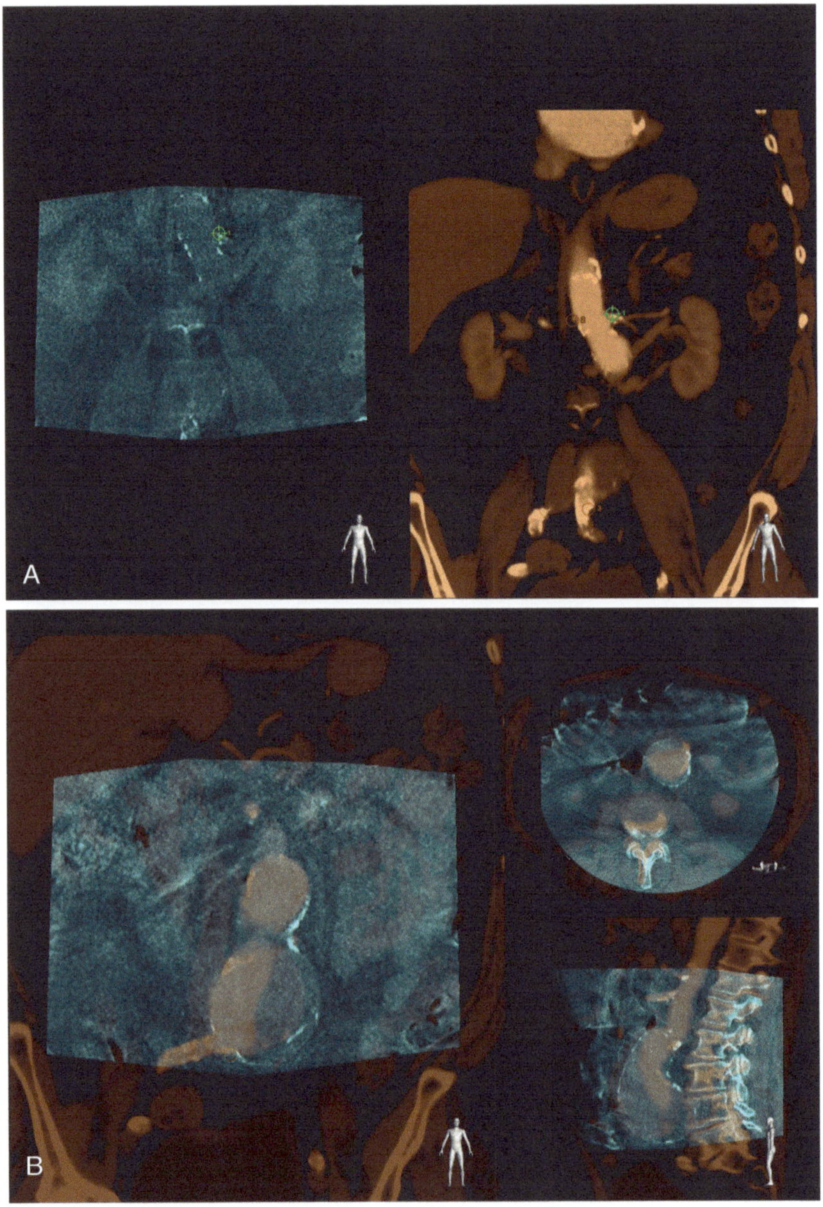

FIG. 20.5 3D/3D registration in fusion imaging. **A,** On the *left,* intraoperative cone-bean CT is shown without contrast agent. On the *right,* preoperative CT angiogram is shown. Based on the calculation, an exact identification of the vessel takeoff is possible, also without contrast agent (points 1, 2, and 3). **B,** The two volumes are overlapped, showing a correct registration.

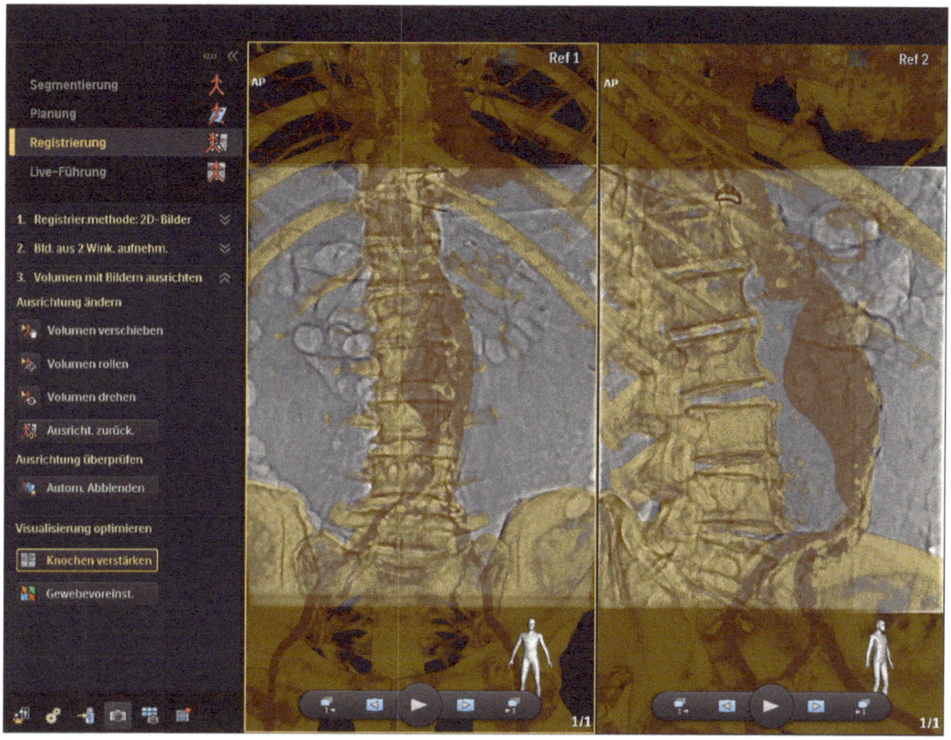

A

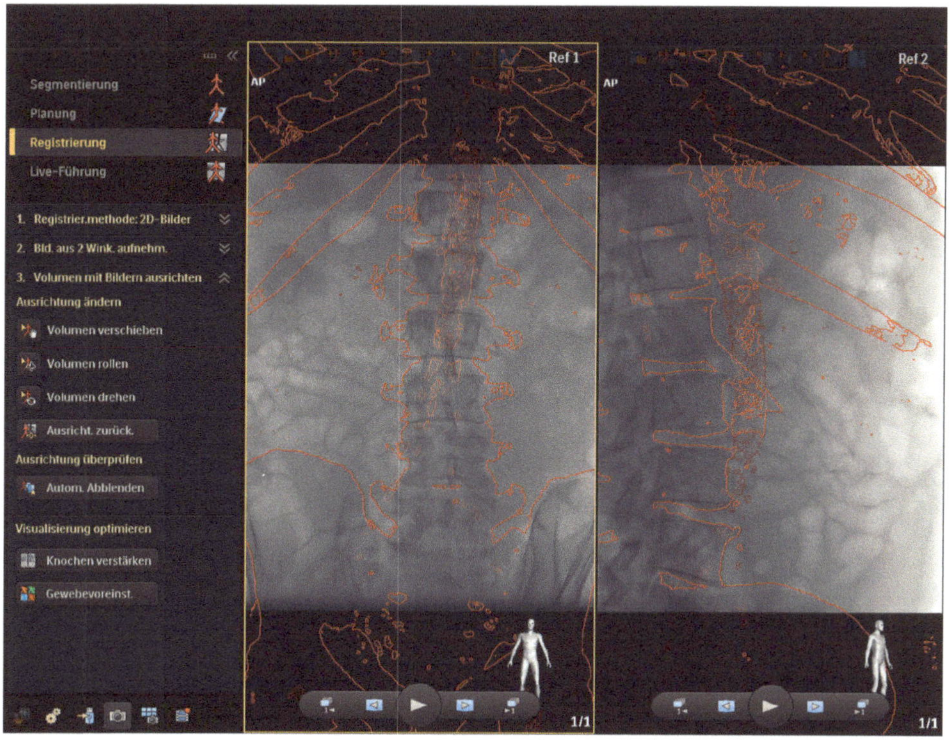

B

FIG. 20.6 **A,** Preoperative volume (*yellow*) is overlayed on the intraoperative 2D images. The bone profiles of the hip and vertebral bodies are emphasized to facilitate merging of the structures. **B,** End of the registration. The *red line* of the intraoperative CT scan follows the profile of the bones.

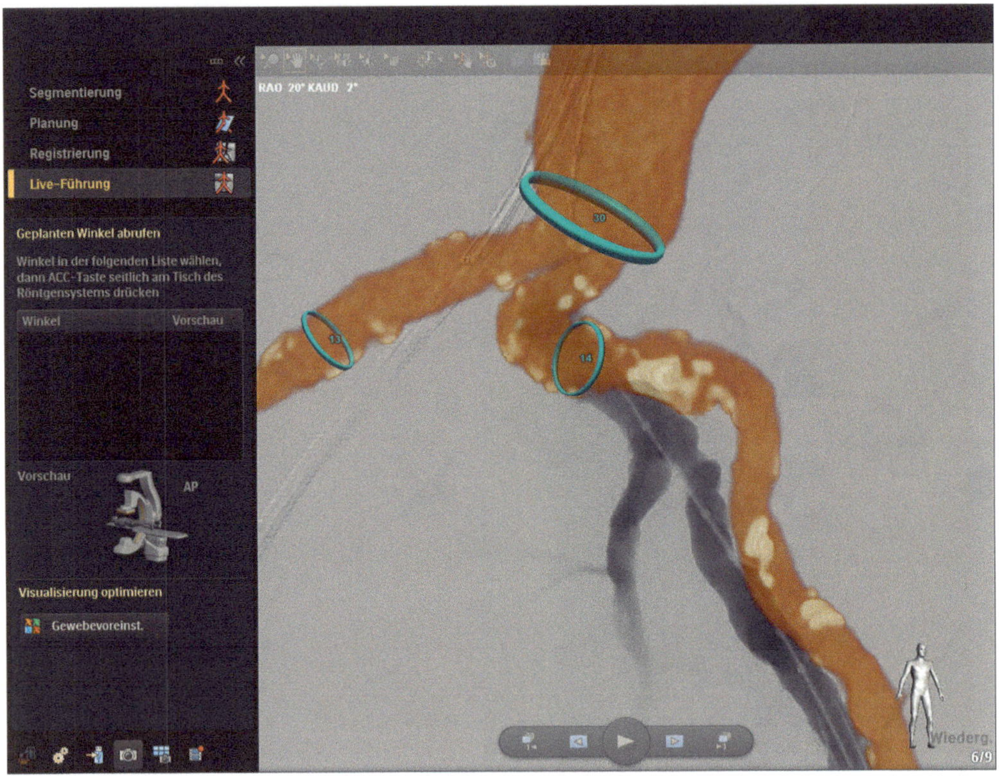

FIG. 20.7 Misalignment at the level of the iliac vessel caused by stiffness of the wire.

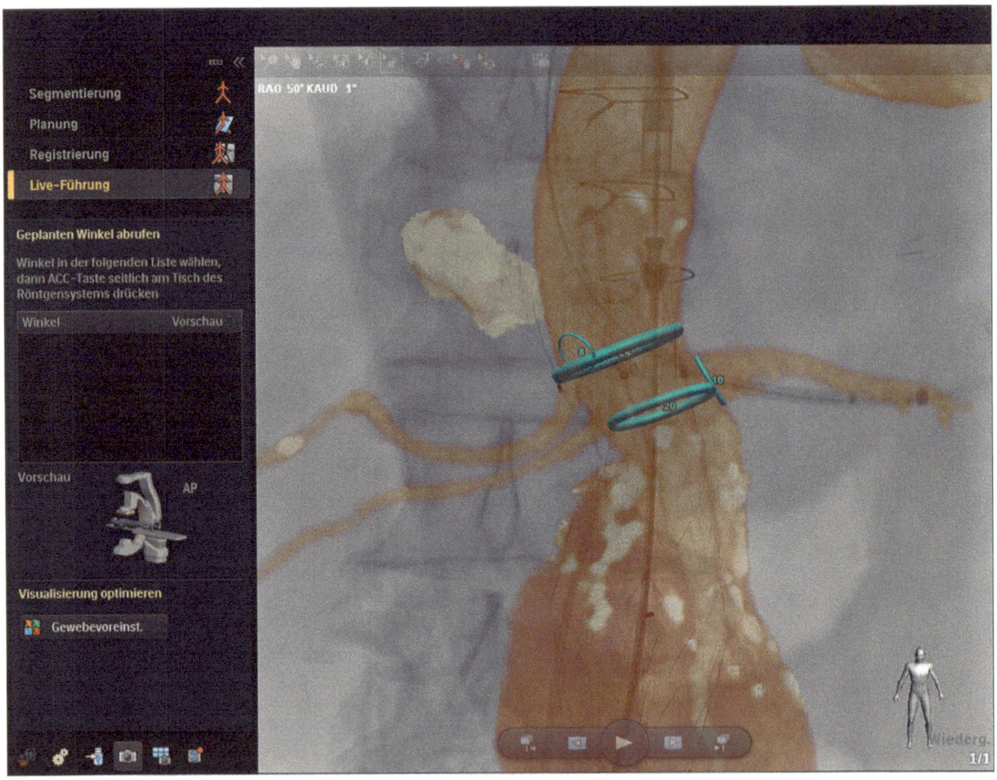

FIG. 20.8 Intraoperative detail during a chimney procedure for the left renal artery. The aortic main body component is deployed just below the takeoff of the main right renal artery. The left renal artery is preserved using a balloon-expandable stent-graft. The accessory renal artery on the right side is intentionally covered.

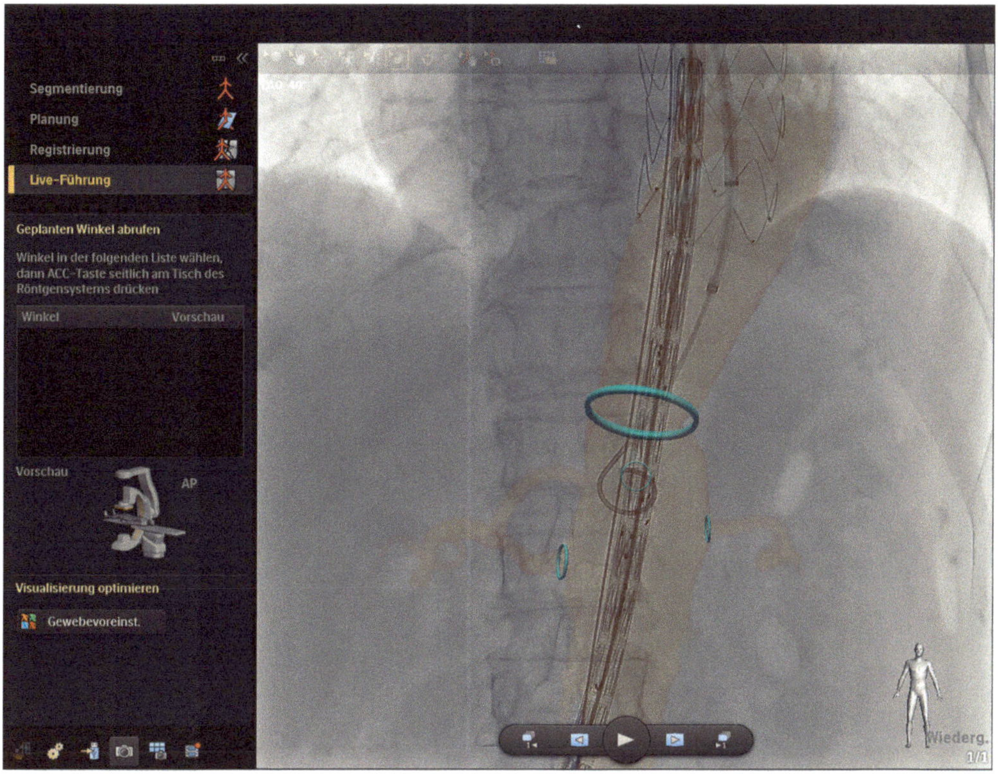

FIG. 20.9 Delivery and deployment of an aortic stent graft, provided by two fenestrations for the renal arteries and one branch for the superior mesenteric artery, assisted by fusion technology.

CONCLUSION

The fusion technique can successfully combine preoperative and intraoperative imaging in aortic procedures. The technique has proved to be feasible and safe. With 2D/3D registration, no additional imaging is needed. The additional information of the 3D volume overlay and markers for vessel origins and landing zone can simplify and shorten complex procedures. Furthermore, it can decrease the amount of contrast agent used and reduce radiation exposure. In most systems the fusion process is fast and simple.

The routine use of fusion imaging techniques is thus an important component in the modern workflow of standard and advanced endovascular aortic aneurysm repair.

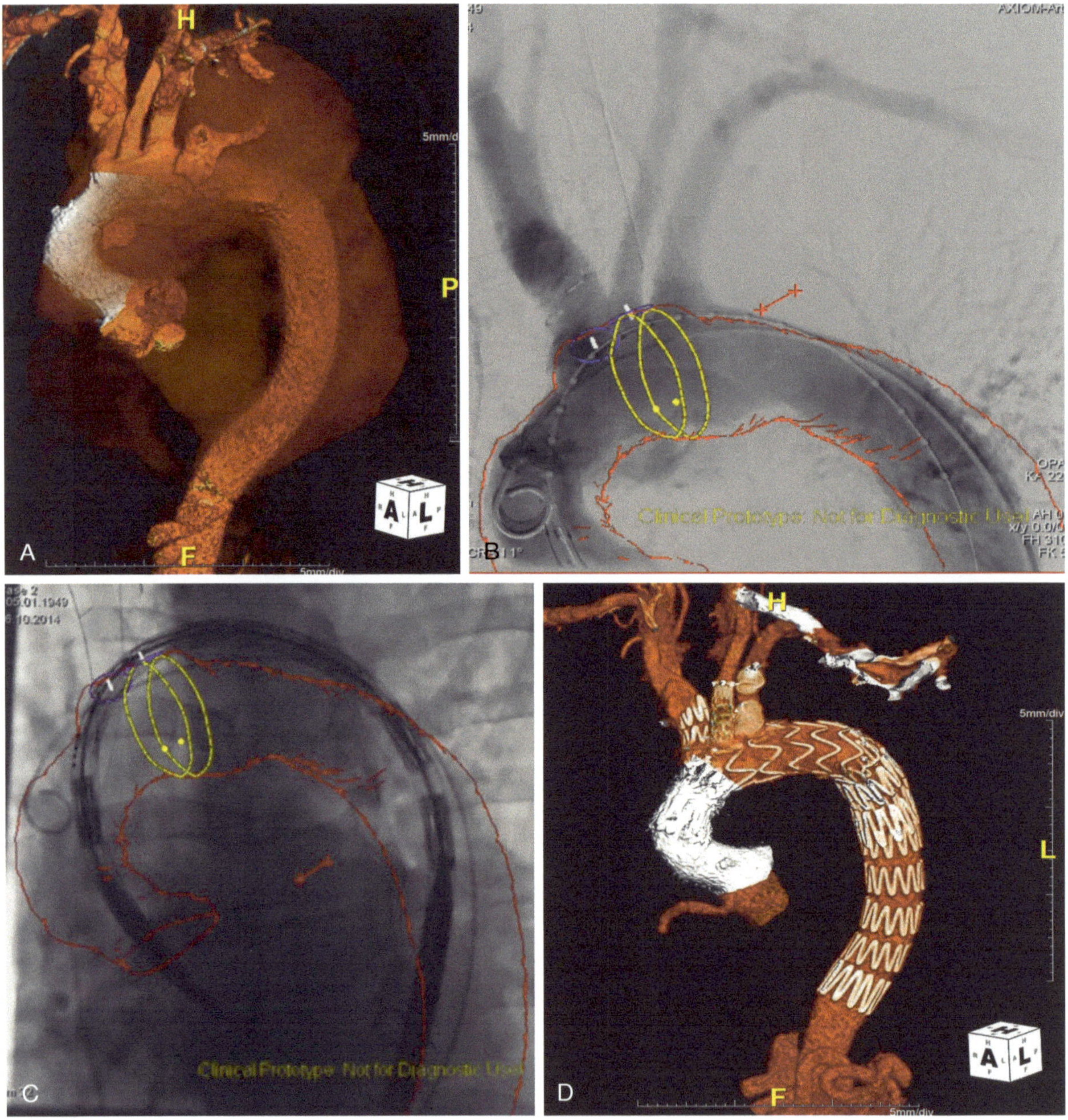

FIG. 20.10 Endovascular treatment of aortic arch aneurysm. **A,** After replacement of the ascending aorta. **B,** Preoperative digital subtraction angiography shows correct registration. **C,** Fusion-assisted graft delivery and deployment. **D,** Postoperative results.

REFERENCES

1. Dijkstra ML, Eagleton MJ, Greenberg RK, Mastracci T, Hernandez A. Intraoperative C-arm cone-beam computed tomography in fenestrated/branched aortic endografting. *J Vasc Surg*. 2011;53:583–590.
2. Panuccio G, Torsello GF, Pfister M, et al. Computer-aided endovascular aortic repair using fully automated two- and three-dimensional fusion imaging. *J Vasc Surg*. 2016;64:1587–1594. e1.
3. Sailer AM, de Haan MW, Peppelenbosch AG, Jacobs MJ, Wildberger JE, Schurink GWH. CTA with fluoroscopy image fusion guidance in endovascular complex aortic aneurysm repair. *Eur J Vasc Endovasc Surg*. 2016;47:349–356.
4. Hertault A, Maurel B, Sobocinski J, et al. Impact of hybrid rooms with image fusion on radiation exposure during endovascular aortic repair. *Eur J Vasc Endovasc Surg*. 2014;48:382–390.

CHAPTER 21

Conclusion and Future Perspectives

KONSTANTINOS P. DONAS

The initial skepticism of endovascular procedures expressed by "traditional" vascular surgeons was replaced with increasing enthusiasm, based on the belief that these less invasive techniques would have an increasingly important role in the treatment of vascular disorders. On the other hand, endovascular complications and durability issues, such as renal impairment caused by contrast medium in follow-up, raised other doubts about endovascular techniques.

Use of endovascular techniques simplifies the treatment of many demanding pathologies that would otherwise be treated by surgical means. The remarkable evolution of the endovascular toolbox expands the application of endovascular aneurysm repair (EVAR) to complex cases. Successful treatment requires clear algorithms that reflect the complementary role of endovascular and open surgical therapeutic modalities. Once the feasibility of these complex endovascular techniques has been demonstrated, the next step is to standardize the techniques and associated devices. In this context, we present in this book the endovascular repair of aortic aneurysms as performed at the Department of Vascular Surgery of St. Franziskus Hospital and University Hospital in Münster, Germany, with standard and advanced techniques.

Durability is the focus of the procedures included in this textbook and will be the focus of future scientific investigation and innovation. The absence of dedicated bridging devices in complex EVAR remains a primary area of interest. In vitro and in vivo testing of the available devices is required. Optimal performance is defined not only by patency but also by the adaptability of the anatomic conditions of the patient. This includes stability of the interaction with the main aortic endografts and the flexibility required by the often-angulated target vessels. These features play a crucial role in the durability of EVAR procedures.

The idea for the present book was born on a ship during a dinner on the Thames River in London. Professor Giovanni Torsello's idea was to present a practical guide for colleagues who perform endovascular repair of aortic aneurysms based on the principles and techniques of the Münster group. I would like to express my deep gratitude to Professor Torsello for his sustained support and a successful 10-year clinical and scientific collaboration.

Index

Note: 'Page numbers followed by "f" indicate figures and "t" indicate tables.'

Kolibri 360 GmbH
Ferdinand-Jühlke-Straße 7
99095 Erfurt, Deutschland
produktsicherheit@kolibri360.de